D0722631

Eating Well to Win

Inspired Living Through Inspired Cooking

Chef RLI Richard Ingraham

FOREWORD BY DWYANE WADE, NBA SUPERSTAR

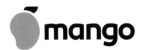 mango

To my parents, Mary and Abe

Thank you for life, love and lessons.
Daddy, I miss you so much.

Foreword

For the past 10 years, Richard Ingraham has been an integral part of my career as an NBA athlete, helping me gain a better understanding of food, health and nutrition. Many probably think the basis of our connections with each other ends there, but what many may not know is that Chef Richard Ingraham—no—Rich is family to me.

Whenever I'm home, you can find Rich in my kitchen preparing meals that help me recover and keep me in shape. When I'm off at practice or traveling, he's holding it down and preparing meals for my wife and three boys in our Chicago home. You see, Rich is not just my guy...he's our guy. It's in the kitchen where you'll find him getting on my boys if they respond and fail to answer with "yes, sir" and "please and thank you." He's there, offering support to my wife and making sure she, too, takes in meals that keep her in great shape while offering support when I'm away on road games. My team members depend on him (sometimes to cater their own private events), and he's loved by everyone in my circle.

And those doggone cookies and red velvet cupcakes; they're too good and get me every time! I'm sure the recipes in the book will have you feeling the same way. Whether you're looking to plan a dinner party with friends and family or cook meals to keep you in shape, Rich will have you covered. Don't just perceive him as an "athlete's chef"...he is a diversified chef that can cook it all, for all. Rich puts his heart and soul into his dishes and I'm so glad he's now found a way to share it with the world!

From my kitchen to yours, Dwyane Wade

Table of Contents

Breakfast

Lunch

Dinner

Dessert

Cover Design: Roberto Núñez
Cover Photo: Bob Metelus
Layout & Design: Nicola DosSantos

For permission requests, please contact the publisher at:
Mango Publishing Group
2850 Douglas Road, 3rd Floor
Coral Gables, FL 33134 USA
info@mango.bz

For special orders, quantity sales, course adoptions and corporate sales, please email the publisher at sales@mango.bz. For trade and wholesale sales, please contact Ingram Publisher Services at customer.service@ingramcontent.com or +1.800.509.4887.

Eating Well To Win: Inspired Living Through Inspired Cooking

Library of Congress Cataloging-in-Publication has been applied for.

ISBN: (hardcover) 978-1- 63353-586- 2, (e-book) 978-1- 63353-587- 9

BISAC category code HEA017000

Printed in the United States of America

Acknowledgements

This book has definitely been a wonderful journey for me to write. I couldn't have done it without the patience, understanding and sacrifice of my wife Stacey (my heart and soul) and my children: Evan, Rj, Kwame and Nandi. Thank you to my business partner, sister and personal bodyguard Soley. Thank you for continuously pushing me to do better. Dwyane and Gabrielle, I can't thank you enough for all of your support and advice over the years. To Team Wade: Lisa, Carmen, Calyann, Bob, Nile, Chantel, Brenda and Lina for being my official taste testers and always having my back. Thank you Marva and the whole Mango Publishing Company for seeing something in me and providing me with the opportunity to write this book.

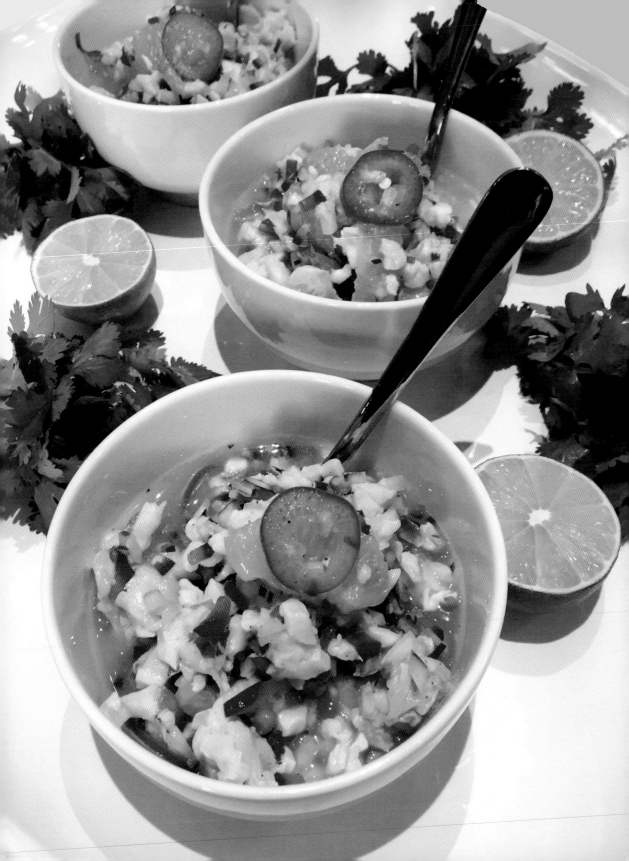

Introduction

Food has always been synonymous to family and love to me.

Cooking a great meal for my friends, family, and clients has become my way of showing them just how much I care about them. This philosophy was instilled in me through witnessing people like my grandmother, my mother, and my uncle put all their love into cooking for our family and friends.

Cooking is such a part of me that I literally dream about what I'm going to cook sometimes. It's not uncommon for me to wake my wife up screaming because I think I'm burning the chicken or something. And, I'm usually up half the night thinking about how I can push myself to cook better than I did the day before.

Being a personal chef is challenging. You're cooking something different three to four times a day almost every day and in my case for up to eight people. So, you have to be self-motivated and constantly educating yourself on new industry trends and ideas. I'm often asked what's my cooking style, and it's the hardest question to answer. I try to dabble in as many different styles as possible to help me create the most memorable experiences for my clients.

I remember when Florida got the lottery back in 1988. It was my senior year in high school, and I vowed that one day I would win! I played a couple of times, but like most, I wasn't successful in my quest to become rich playing this game of chance.

It wasn't until years later, as I walked into Dwyane and Gabrielle's home and started my usual routine of turning on the ovens and stoves, making my essential cup of coffee and plotting out what I'm going to create for the day that I began looking around and looking back on how I got here. How is it that I'm doing something that I love doing every single day? How did I make it to this point? Just then, I realized that I had done what I set out to do back in 1988. I had truly won the lottery!!!

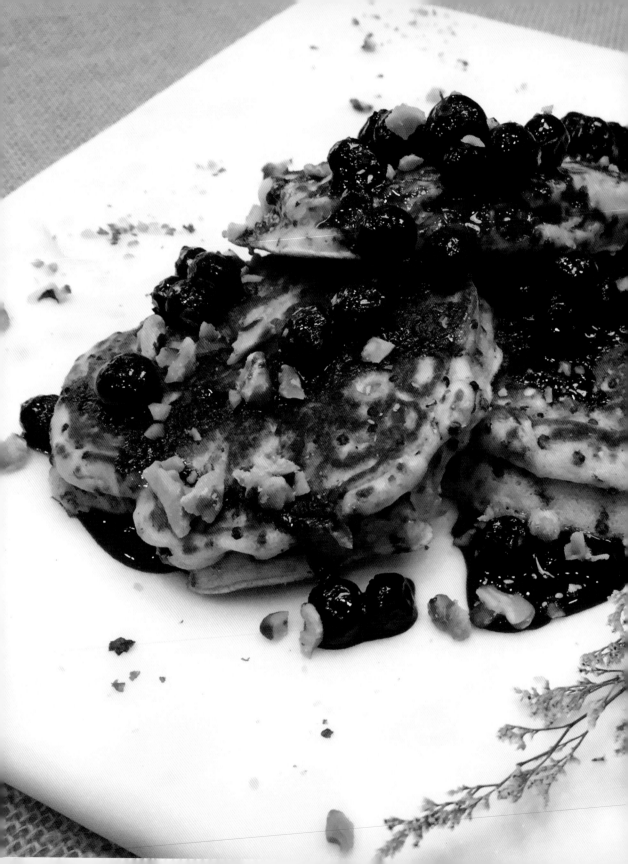

Breakfast

As a child, I remember waking up to the smells and sounds of breakfast being cooked. It didn't matter what happened the day before. Waking up to my mother's breakfast was my automatic reset button for a new day.

Breakfast is important not only for your body but for your mind as well. Whether you're sitting down with maple syrup drizzled warm cinnamon pancakes, sausage, and fluffy scrambled eggs or you've got just enough time to get a green smoothie from the local juice bar, it starts your day, provides you with energy, and makes you happy.

That happiness leads to a smile and a good morning to someone you don't even know, which in turn leads them to do the same to someone else. So, you see, breakfast is also great for your soul.

Eating Breakfast to Win

Eating a nutritious breakfast helps you kick-start your metabolism. By starting your day with lean protein, whole grains and healthy fats, you'll be energized and less likely to reach for comfort snacks later in the day.

Caribbean Salmon Croquettes with Cilantro Aioli

For Croquettes

2 cans of pink salmon, drained

½ cup red onion, minced

2 teaspoons Creole seasoning

½ teaspoon garlic powder

½ teaspoon cumin

½ teaspoon smoked paprika

3 tablespoons fresh, chopped cilantro

¼ cup red bell pepper, diced small

1 ½ tablespoons Dijon mustard

½ cup asiago cheese

¾ cup gluten free panko
bread crumbs

2 large eggs, beaten

½ cup of canola or vegetable oil

For Cilantro Aioli

½ cup fresh cilantro, chopped

1 lime, juiced

1 teaspoon ground cumin

1 cup avocado mayonnaise

2 cloves garlic, minced

2 teaspoons honey

Salt and pepper

Cilantro Aioli

1. Combine all ingredients in a blender, and mix until well incorporated.

2. Adjust seasonings, and serve.

Croquettes

1. In a large bowl, gently break apart the salmon.

2. Add the remainder of the ingredients except the oil.

3. To test flavor of salmon mixture: Heat oil in a skillet over medium-high heat and carefully add a tablespoon of the salmon mixture shaped into a patty. Since the mix has raw egg in it, you can't taste it beforehand. This gives you a chance to test the flavor before you make the rest of your croquettes.

4. Cook until browned. Use a fish spatula to carefully turn and brown the other side.

5. Drain on paper towel, taste and adjust seasoning.

6. Form the rest of the mixture into patties, and resume the cooking process.

7. Serve immediately with cilantro aioli.

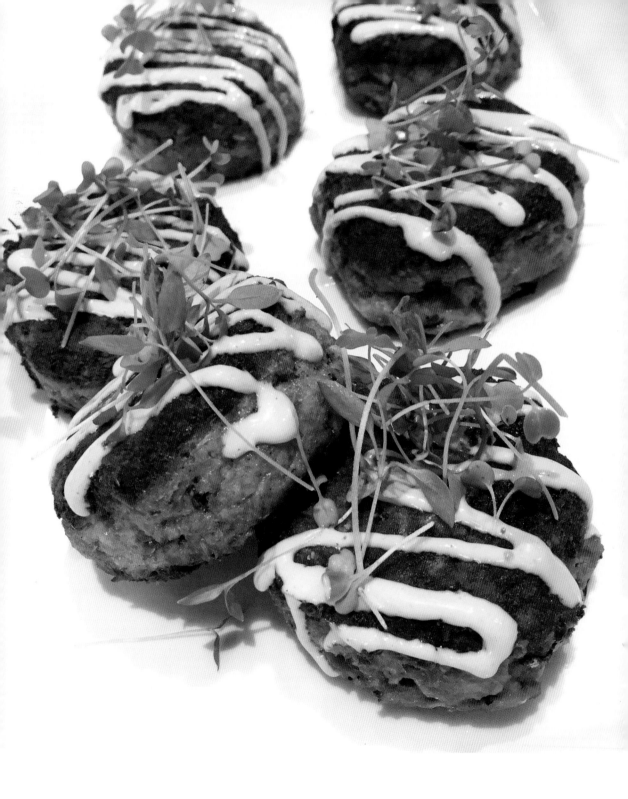

Crab and Mushroom Frittata

2 tablespoons olive oil, divided

1 medium shallot

8 ounces velvet pioppini mushrooms
(any other mushroom will work just
as well)

¼ cup smoked, sun-dried tomatoes

½ cup lump crabmeat

1 avocado, diced

12 large eggs

½ cup heavy cream

¾ cup shredded asiago cheese, divided

Kosher salt and freshly ground pepper

1. Preheat your oven to 350 degrees.

2. Heat one tablespoon of oil in a nonstick ovenproof skillet over medium heat.

3. Add shallots, and stir until softened.

4. Add mushrooms and stir often until softened and all liquid has been released.

5. In a large bowl, whisk eggs, cream and ½ cup cheese.

6. Season with salt and pepper.

7. Add crab, avocado and tomatoes to the skillet.

8. Increase the heat to medium high, and add remaining tablespoon of oil to the skillet.

9. Pour the egg mixture over the mushrooms, and shake to make sure the eggs are evenly distributed.

10. Cook without stirring, until it's set. This should take about five minutes.

11. Sprinkle remaining ¼ cup cheese over eggs, and transfer skillet to oven.

12. Bake frittata until golden brown and center is set.

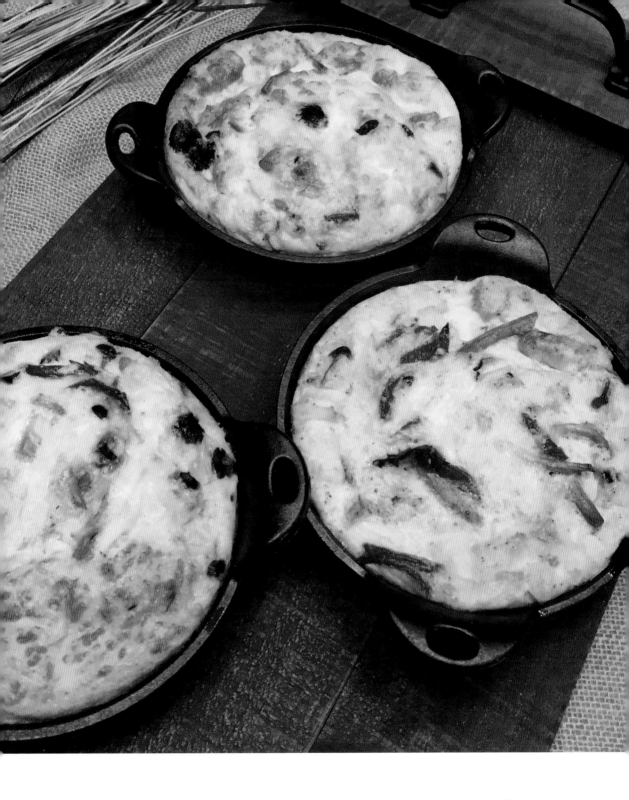

Spicy Lobster and Sweet Potato Grits

For Lobster

1 tablespoon grape seed oil

4 ounces turkey andouille sausage, sliced

1 ½ teaspoons Creole seasoning

2 medium lobster tails, split and meat completely removed and chopped from one tail

1 tablespoon unsalted butter

1 medium shallot, minced

3 garlic cloves, thinly sliced

1 tablespoon celery, minced

1 ½ teaspoons crushed red pepper flakes

1 cup fire-roasted tomatoes

1 teaspoon Worcestershire sauce

2 teaspoons fresh thyme

Kosher salt and fresh ground pepper

For Grits

1 tablespoon unsalted butter

¼ cup onions, chopped

4 cups chicken broth

1 teaspoon Creole seasoning

½ teaspoon cinnamon

¼ teaspoon nutmeg

1 cup uncooked yellow grits

1 cup heavy cream

2 tablespoons butter

1 sweet potato, roasted and mashed

½ cup smoked Gouda cheese

Lobster

1. Heat oil in a large sauté pan over medium heat, and brown sausage turning frequently to ensure even cooking.

2. Remove sausage from the pan using a slotted spoon, and drain on a paper-towel lined baking pan.

3. Pour out all but ½ tablespoon of oil from the pan, and return to the stove over medium heat.

4. Raise the temperature of the pan to medium-high heat, and add lobster to the pan.

5. Cook lobster just enough so that it begins to brown.

6. Remove lobster from the pan, place in a bowl and reserve.

7. Return the pan to the stove, and reduce the heat to medium.

8. Add butter to the pan.

9. Once the butter starts to foam, add in the shallots, garlic, celery and red pepper flakes.

10. Stir often until the mixture is slightly softened.

11. Add fire-roasted tomatoes and Worcestershire sauce.

12. Stir until tomatoes begin to release their juices. This normally takes about five minutes.

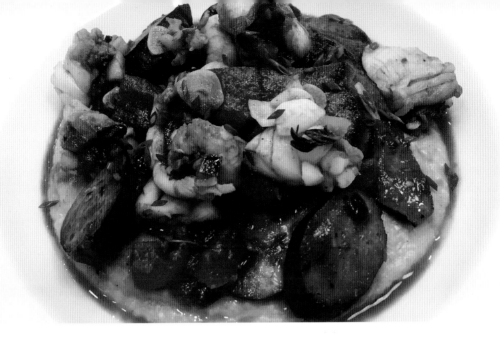

13. Add reserved lobster and sausage to the pan, and cook until lobster is warmed through.

14. Add fresh time, and adjust seasonings.

Method for Grits

1. Melt one tablespoon of butter in a medium saucepot over medium heat.

2. Add onions, and stir often until onions soften.

3. Pour in broth and bring to a boil over high heat.

4. Once broth reaches a rolling boil, pour in the grits. Whisk the grits as you pour them in to prevent lumps.

5. Add in cinnamon, Creole seasoning and nutmeg.

6. Stir the grits until the mixture comes back up to a boil, then reduce the heat to low.

7. Place a lid on top, and let simmer.

8. Combine the mashed sweet potato and cream in a medium bowl, and mix into a puree.

9. After the grits have cooked, remove the lid and stir in the sweet potato mixture until well blended.

10. Finish by adding the butter and smoked Gouda.

11. Taste and adjust seasonings. Spoon over the lobster, and serve hot.

Crab and Vegetable Scramble Avocado Toast

6 large eggs

1 ½ tablespoons heavy cream

¼ cup white cheddar cheese

2 tablespoons unsalted butter

½ small red onion, minced

½ red bell pepper small, diced

6 asparagus, chopped

2 garlic cloves, minced

2 tablespoons cilantro, chopped

8 ounces lump crabmeat, picked
   for shells

1 teaspoon cumin

Kosher salt and freshly ground pepper

4 large slices country-style bread,
   toasted (any type of bread will
   work just fine)

3 avocados, halved, pitted, peeled
   and sliced

Sriracha

1. In a large bowl, whisk together eggs, cream, salt, pepper and cheese, and set to the side.

2. In a large heavy nonstick skillet over medium-low heat, melt butter.

3. Add vegetables and sauté until slightly softened.

4. Add crab to vegetables.

5. Pour in egg mixture and season with salt, pepper and cumin.

6. Occasionally scrape bottom of skillet with a heatproof spatula to form large, soft curds. Then cook until desired firmness is achieved. Set aside.

7. Place two slices of toast on each plate.

8. Place slices of avocado on each slice of bread, then top with the eggs.

9. Drizzle Sriracha, and serve immediately.

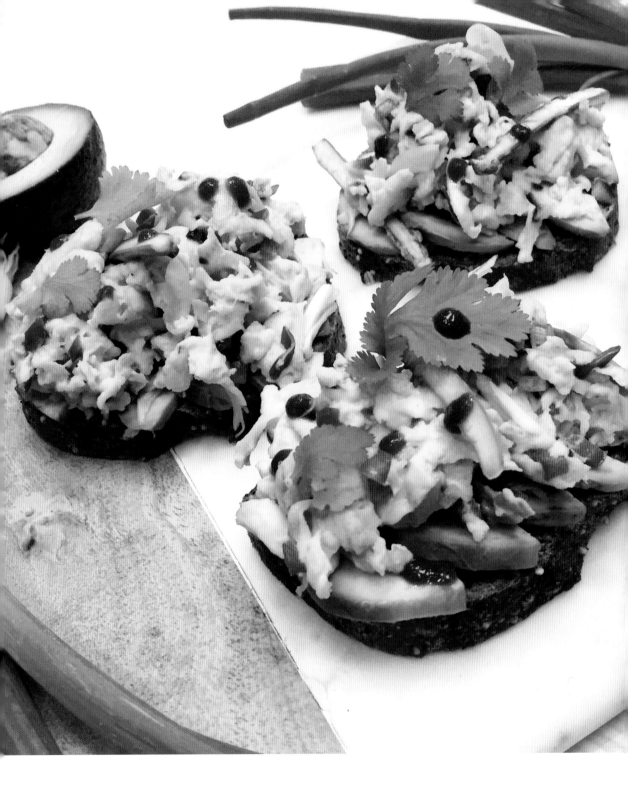

Smoked Salmon and Avocado Toast

4 pieces country-style bread, toasted
 (any type of bread will work just fine)

2 small avocados, peeled, pitted

1 small lemon, juiced

½ small red onion, minced

1 tablespoon fresh dill, chopped

 Kosher salt and freshly ground pepper

8 ounces smoked salmon

1 teaspoon fresh chives, chopped

¼ cup microgreens

1 teaspoon lemon zest

1 teaspoon olive oil

1. Place avocado in a medium bowl, and smash with the back of a fork until fairly smooth.

2. Stir in lemon juice, onion, ½ tablespoon dill, and season with salt and pepper.

3. In a separate bowl, combine chives, microgreens, zest, ½ tablespoon dill and olive oil.

4. Gently stir to incorporate, and season with salt and pepper.

5. Spread avocado onto each slice, and top each with two ounces of smoked salmon.

6. Finish by topping toast with microgreen salad. Serve immediately.

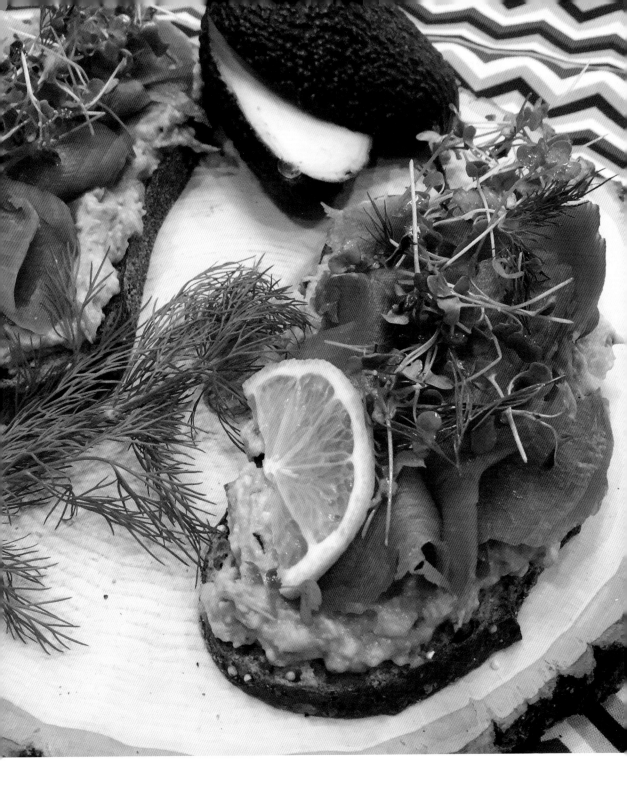

Collard Green and Mushroom Toast with Eggplant Puree

For Toast

2 cups wild mushrooms (Any combination will work, but I'm a fan of velvet pioppini, brown clamshell and forest nameko.)

3 garlic cloves, sliced thin

¼ medium red onion, sliced thin

2 teaspoons grape seed oil

2 cups collard greens, large stems removed and leaves torn

1 tablespoon fig balsamic vinegar

Kosher salt and freshly ground pepper

Country-style bread, toasted (any type of bread will work just fine)

For Eggplant Puree

2 medium eggplants

8 cloves garlic

Kosher salt and freshly ground pepper

2 tablespoons olive oil

1 teaspoon smoked paprika

Eggplant

1. Preheat your oven to 375 degrees.

2. Split the eggplants lengthwise.

3. Using a paring knife create two slits in each eggplant half. You should have eight slits in all.

4. Place 1 clove of garlic in each slit.

5. Coat the white flesh of all the eggplants with olive oil, and season with salt and pepper.

6. Place each half of eggplant on a baking sheet, cut side down.

7. Bake until the flesh is soft and the skin has no resistance when poked with a knife.

8. Remove from oven and allow to cool until you can handle them.

9. Scrape the flesh away from the skin into a blender or food processor, making sure all the garlic is included.

10. Season eggplant with paprika, salt and pepper.

11. Blend until smooth and creamy.

12. Adjust seasoning, and reserve until ready to be used.

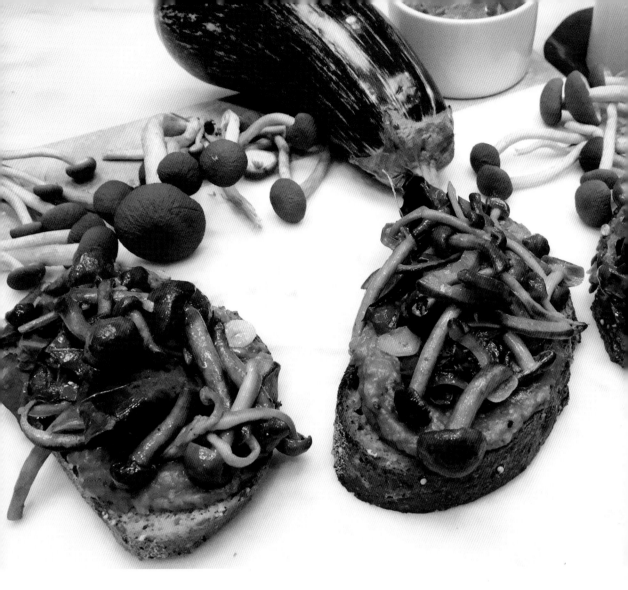

Toast

1. In a large sauté pan over medium-high heat, cook mushrooms, garlic and onions in grape seed oil until browned and most of the moisture is removed from the mushrooms.

2. Add greens, and cook until wilted.

3. Season mixture with vinegar, salt and pepper, and remove from the heat.

4. Spread eggplant puree onto toasted bread.

5. Top eggplant puree with spoon mushroom mixture, and serve immediately.

Collard Green Ham and Smoked Gouda Strata

3 cups collard greens, large stems
   removed and leaves chopped

3 tablespoons olive oil

1 large red onion, diced

1 red bell pepper, seeded and diced

4 cloves garlic, sliced

1 teaspoon Creole seasoning

1 teaspoon freshly ground pepper

8 cups whole wheat country bread,
   cut into 1-inch cubes

2 cups smoked Gouda cheese

1 cup diced ham

8 large eggs

3 cups unsweetened almond milk

1 tablespoon Dijon mustard

1 teaspoon curry powder

2 teaspoons fresh thyme

1. Preheat the oven to 350 degrees.

2. Butter a 9-by-12-inch baking dish.

3. Heat oil in a large skillet over medium heat, and sauté the onion, peppers and garlic until soft.

4. Add the collard greens, Creole seasoning and pepper.

5. Cook until the greens are wilted then remove from heat.

6. Spread half the bread cubes in the prepared baking dish.

7. Top with half the collard green mixture.

8. Sprinkle with half the ham and half the cheese.

9. Repeat this process ending with cheese.

10. In a medium bowl, whisk together the eggs, almond milk, mustard, curry, Creole seasoning and thyme until well incorporated.

11. Pour the custard evenly over the strata, and cover with plastic wrap and refrigerate overnight.

12. Remove the strata from the fridge, and let it come to room temperature.

13. Bake the strata uncovered until golden brown and cooked through.

14. Cut into squares, and serve from the same baking dish with sliced green onions for garnish.

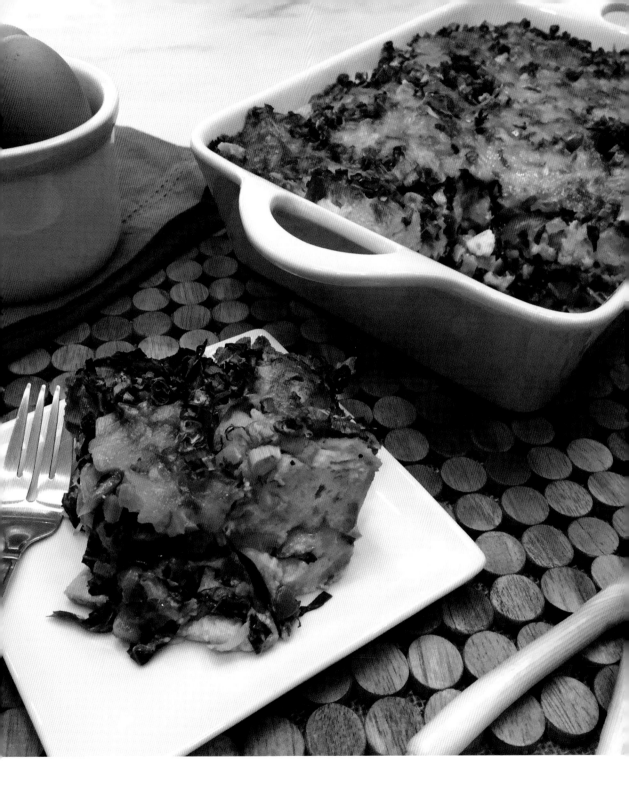

Pear Dutch Baby with Blackberry St. Germain Syrup

For Dutch Baby

3 tablespoons unsalted butter

2 ripe pears, cored and
   sliced ¼ inch thick

6 tablespoons maple syrup

1 teaspoon ground cinnamon

2 large eggs

½ cup unsweetened vanilla almond milk

½ cup white, whole-wheat flour

1 teaspoon bourbon vanilla extract

¼ teaspoon salt

⅛ teaspoon ground nutmeg

For Blackberry Syrup

4 cups blackberries

¾ cup maple syrup

¼ cup water

¼ St. Germain (elderflower liquor)

Confectioners' sugar, for dusting

Lemon wedges, for serving

Dutch Baby

1. Preheat your oven to 450 degrees.

2. In a medium skillet over medium heat, melt two tablespoons butter.

3. Add the pears, four tablespoons maple syrup and ½ teaspoon cinnamon, and cook until the pears are caramelized and tender. Remove from the heat, and reserve in the pan.

4. Place two tablespoons of butter in a 10-inch, cast-iron skillet and place in the oven until the butter is melted and the skillet is very hot.

5. In a blender, mix together the eggs, almond milk, whole-wheat flour, the remaining two tablespoons of maple syrup, the remaining ½ teaspoon of the cinnamon, vanilla, salt and nutmeg until smooth.

6. Pour batter into a medium bowl. Using a slotted spoon, remove half of the caramelized pears, and fold them into the batter.

7. Carefully pour the batter into the pre-heated skillet, and place it in the oven.

8. Bake until the edges of the pancake are golden brown and have puffed up.

9. Once the Dutch baby is removed from the oven, top with the remaining caramelized pears, and dust with powdered sugar.

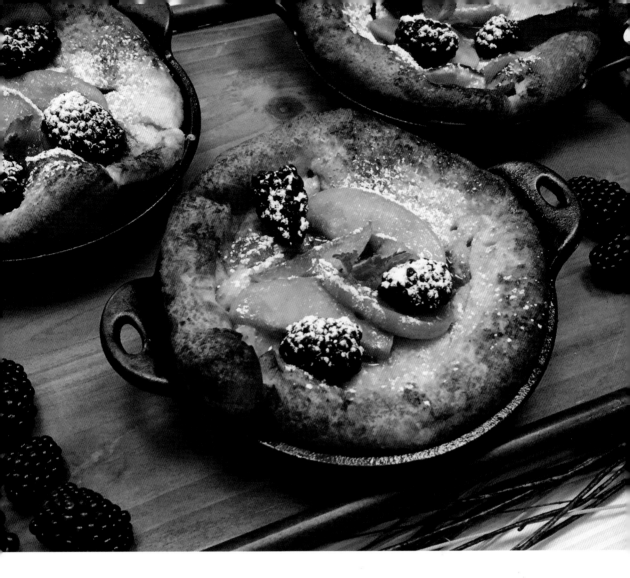

Blackberry Syrup

1. In a medium saucepan over medium heat, combine berries, sugar, water and St. Germain.

2. Bring mixture to a boil, stirring until sugar is dissolved.

3. Reduce heat to medium, and simmer until blackberries are soft.

4. Pour syrup through a fine-mesh sieve into a bowl, pressing gently on the blackberries and then discarding solids.

5. Serve syrup warm over the Dutch baby.

Cheddar and Chive Cornbread Waffles with Curry Fried Chicken

For Waffles

1 ½ cups coarse cornmeal

¾ cup white, whole-wheat flour

3 teaspoons baking powder

2 teaspoons baking soda

2 teaspoons Creole seasoning

1 ½ teaspoons smoked paprika

1 ½ teaspoons garlic powder

½ cup grated, smoked cheddar

¼ cup chives, chopped

2 tablespoons honey

2 cups buttermilk

½ tablespoon hot sauce

2 eggs

1 stick unsalted butter, melted

For Chicken

2 pounds chicken wings (drumsticks or thighs are okay, but I'm a wing man)

1 ½ tablespoons Creole seasoning

2 ½ tablespoons curry powder

1 ½ teaspoons dried thyme

1 teaspoon black pepper

2 large eggs

¼ cup buttermilk

2 cups all-purpose flour (regular all-purpose flour is my go-to for frying chicken)

½ tablespoon curry powder

½ tablespoon dried thyme

Canola oil for frying

For Corn Relish

5 ears of sweet yellow corn, kernels sliced off the cob

1 large red bell pepper, finely chopped

1 large orange bell pepper, finely chopped

3 stalks celery, chopped

2 jalapeños, seeded and finely chopped

1 medium yellow onion, finely chopped

2 cups apple cider vinegar

1 cup sugar

½ teaspoon ground dry mustard

2 teaspoons Kosher salt

Chicken

1. In a small bowl, combine Creole seasoning, curry, thyme and black pepper.

2. Season wings with the spice mixture.

3. In a large bowl, beat the eggs and buttermilk together.

4. In a separate bowl, whisk together the flour and ½ tablespoon of Creole seasoning, curry and thyme.

5. Dredge the chicken in the egg and buttermilk mixture then dredge in the flour.

6. Shake off any excess flour. Place the coated pieces aside on a wire rack, and repeat with the remaining chicken.

7. Fill a fryer with oil, and heat to 350 degrees.

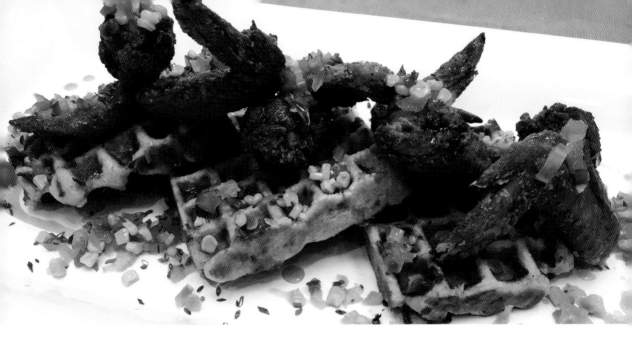

8. Fry the chicken wings until they are crispy, begin to float and juices run clear. This usually takes about 10 minutes.

Relish

1. In a medium pot over medium-high heat, combine all the ingredients and bring to a boil, continuously stirring until the sugar is dissolved.

2. Reduce the heat to medium, and simmer uncovered until the vegetables are tender.

3. Remove relish from the heat, and let fully cool before use.

Waffles

1. Preheat waffle iron.

2. In a large bowl, combine cornmeal, flour, baking powder, baking soda, one tablespoon Creole seasoning, paprika, garlic powder, cheddar and chives.

3. In a separate bowl, beat together eggs, buttermilk, honey, hot sauce and melted butter.

4. Make a well in the center of the dry ingredients, and stir in the buttermilk mixture until just combined.

5. Brush both sides of your waffle iron with butter, and add 1/3 cup of the batter into the center of your iron. Close and cook until nicely browned.

6. Top waffles with curry fried chicken, corn relish and maple syrup.

Sweet Potato Waffles with Caramelized Bananas

For Waffles

- 3 cups white, whole-wheat flour
- 2 tablespoons baking powder
- 1 teaspoon salt
- 1½ teaspoons cinnamon
- 1 teaspoon nutmeg
- ½ teaspoon kosher salt
- 1 teaspoon ground ginger
- 2 cups buttermilk
- ¼ cup maple syrup
- 1 cup sour cream
- 1 teaspoon bourbon vanilla extract
- 1 cup mashed, baked sweet potatoes
- 1 stick unsalted butter, melted
- 3 large eggs, room temperature
- 2 medium bananas, chopped

For Bananas

- 3 firm, ripe bananas
- 2 tablespoons butter, melted
- 2 tablespoons brown sugar
- 2 tablespoons spiced rum
- ½ teaspoon cinnamon

Waffles

1. Pre-heat your waffle iron.

2. Combine all of the dry ingredients in a large bowl, and whisk until well combined.

3. Separate the egg yolks from the whites, and place them in separate bowls.

4. In a medium bowl, combine the milk, sour cream, mashed sweet potato, melted butter, egg yolks and vanilla.

5. Whisk until well combined.

6. Using an electric stand mixer or a hand mixer, beat the egg whites at a high speed until stiff peaks form.

7. Pour the wet ingredients over the dry ingredients, and mix until just combined being careful not to over mix.

8. Fold in the beaten egg whites.

9. Coat waffle iron with nonstick spray. Working in batches, add batter to waffle iron. The amount needed and cooking time will vary depending on the machine.

10. Sprinkle about four to five pieces of chopped banana on top of each waffle before closing iron.

11. Cook until waffles are lightly browned and set.

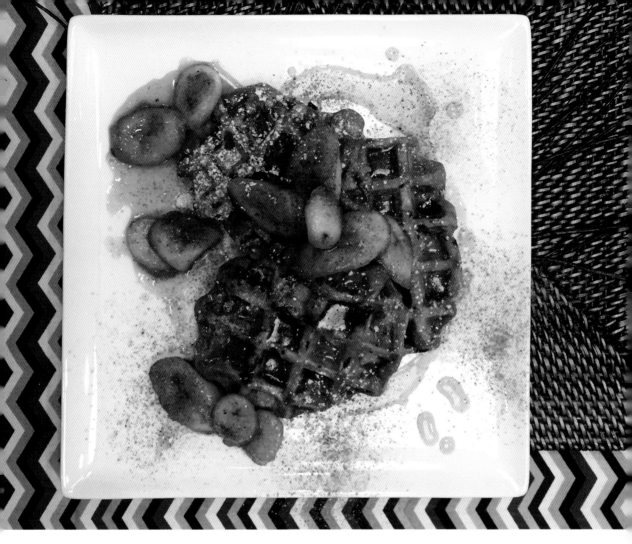

Bananas

1. Cut bananas in half lengthwise.

2. Melt butter in a nonstick skillet over medium-high heat.

3. Add brown sugar, and lay banana slices on top, cut side up.

4. Cook bananas for about 20 to 25 seconds. (You will want to check on them, but resist the urge and leave them alone.)

5. Next add rum and cinnamon.

6. Carefully turn bananas, and cook for another 40 seconds basting with the rum caramel sauce.

7. Remove from heat, and immediately place on top of waffles.

S'mores Pancakes

For Pancakes

2 cups white, whole-wheat flour

2 teaspoons baking powder

1 teaspoon baking soda

4 tablespoons cacao powder (this is a healthier option than cocoa)

1 teaspoon salt

1 ½ teaspoons bourbon vanilla extract

2 tablespoons maple syrup

2 cups buttermilk

²/₃ cup mini chocolate chips

1 cup medium marshmallows

1 sheet graham crackers, crushed

Special Equipment: kitchen torch for marshmallows

For Chocolate Syrup

2 cups honey

1 cup cacao powder

2 cups water

1 teaspoon bourbon vanilla extract

¼ teaspoon salt

Chocolate Syrup

1. Pour honey, cacao, water and salt into a medium saucepan, and cook over high heat stirring until dissolved.

2. Bring mixture to a boil.

3. Lower heat to medium, and simmer, stirring constantly.

4. When the syrup reaches the desired thickness, remove from heat, and stir in vanilla.

5. Allow syrup to cool before use.

Pancakes

1. Place marshmallows on a parchment paper lined baking sheet. Ignite the torch and move steadily back and forth over the surface of the marshmallow topping until it's toasted to your satisfaction. If your parchment paper flames up, move the torch and blow out the fire. Reserve until ready to use.

2. Combine all dry ingredients in a medium bowl, and mix well.

3. In a separate bowl, combine all wet ingredients.

4. Make a well in the dry ingredients and pour in the liquid ingredients. Mix just until combined.

5. Fold in chocolate chips.

6. Pour ¼ cup of the pancake batter onto a hot, lightly oiled griddle.

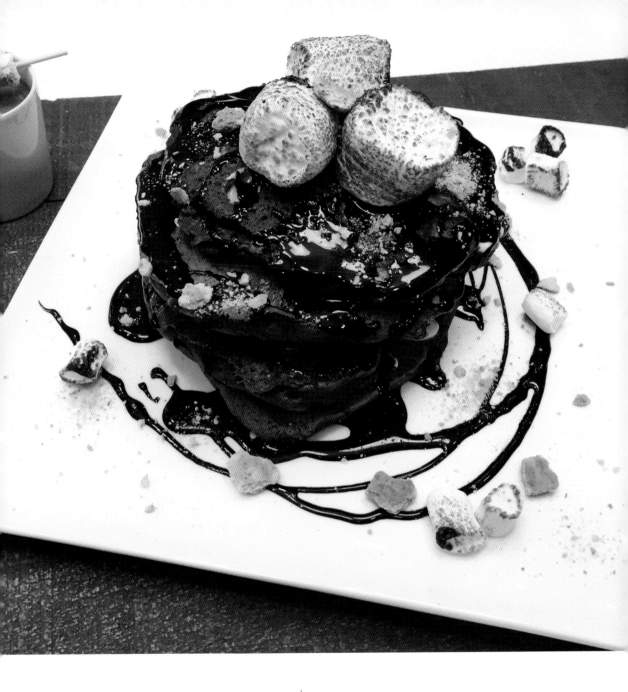

7. Cook for one to two minutes then flip pancakes once air bubbles begin to rise to the surface.

8. Plate hot pancakes, and garnish with graham crackers, toasted marshmallows and chocolate sauce.

Blueberry Poppy Seed Pancakes with Lemon Crème Fraîche

For Pancakes

2 cups white, whole-wheat flour

2 teaspoons baking powder

1 ½ teaspoons baking soda

1 teaspoon salt

Zest of 2 lemons

4 tablespoons poppy seeds

2 cups fresh blueberries

2 whole eggs

1 ½ teaspoons bourbon vanilla extract

¼ cup maple syrup

2 cups unsweetened,
   vanilla almond milk

1 tablespoon lemon juice

For Lemon Crème Fraîche

¼ cup crème fraîche (you can
   substitute sour cream)

½ teaspoon fresh lemon juice

¼ teaspoon finely grated lemon zest

1 teaspoon honey

Creme Fraîche

1. Combine crème fraîche, lemon juice, lemon zest and honey in small bowl.

Pancakes

1. Combine all dry ingredients (use only 1 ½ cups of the blueberries) in a medium bowl, and mix well.

2. In a separate bowl, combine all wet ingredients.

3. Make a well in the dry ingredients, and pour in the liquid ingredients. Mix just until combined.

4. Pour ¼ cup of the pancake batter onto a hot, lightly oiled griddle.

5. Cook for one to two minutes then flip pancakes once air bubbles begin to rise to the surface.

6. Plate hot pancakes, garnish with lemon crème fraîche and ½ cup of fresh blueberries.

7. Serve with maple syrup.

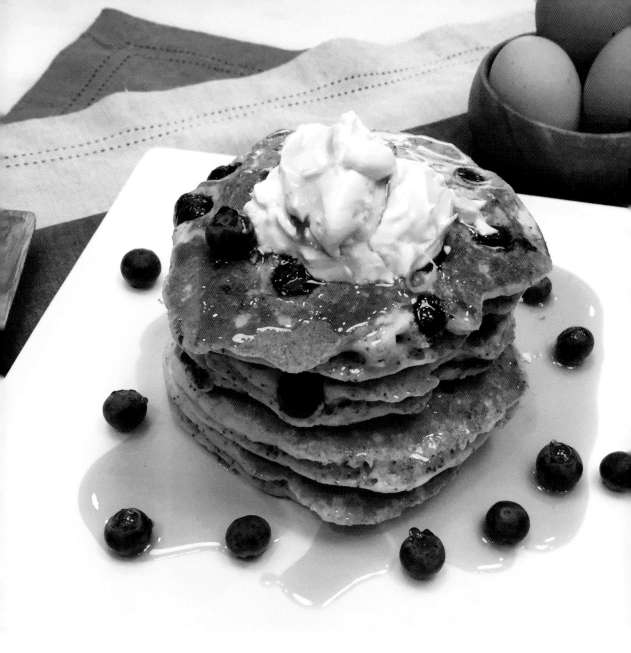

Bonus:

To take this dish to another level, try combining ½ cup of maple syrup with two cups of blueberries in a small pot over medium heat and simmer until berries are softened, then mash the berries using the back of a spoon. Remove syrup from heat, strain out the solids and stir in ½ cup fresh blueberries and the zest from one lemon. Use this to top your pancakes.

Buckwheat Pancakes with Maple Apples

For Pancakes

2 cups buckwheat flour

1/2 cup oat flour (you can make your own by putting 1 cup of whole-wheat, old-fashioned oats in a blender on high until it becomes a fine powder)

2 tablespoons maple syrup

2 teaspoons baking powder

1/2 teaspoon baking soda

2 teaspoons cinnamon

1 teaspoon ground ginger

1/2 teaspoon salt

2 large eggs

1 1/2 teaspoons bourbon vanilla extract

2 cups buttermilk

For Maple Apples

2 tablespoons unsalted butter

2 Granny Smith apples, peeled and sliced

1/4 cup pure maple syrup

1 teaspoon cinnamon

1/4 teaspoon cloves

1/4 teaspoon salt

Maple Apples

1. Brown apples in butter in a medium pan over medium heat.

2. Once browned, add in maple syrup, cinnamon, cloves and salt.

3. Reduce heat to low, and simmer until apples are soft.

Pancakes

1. Combine all dry ingredients in a medium bowl, and mix to fully incorporate.

2. In a separate bowl, combine all wet ingredients, and mix to fully incorporate.

3. Make a well in the day ingredients, and pour in the buttermilk mixture.

4. Mix the two just until they are combined, careful not to over mix. If the batter is over mixed, your pancakes won't be tender and fluffy.

5. Pour 1/4 cup of the pancake batter onto a hot, lightly oiled griddle.

6. Cook for one to two minutes then flip pancakes once air bubbles begin to rise to the surface.

7. Plate hot pancakes, and serve with maple apples as a garnish.

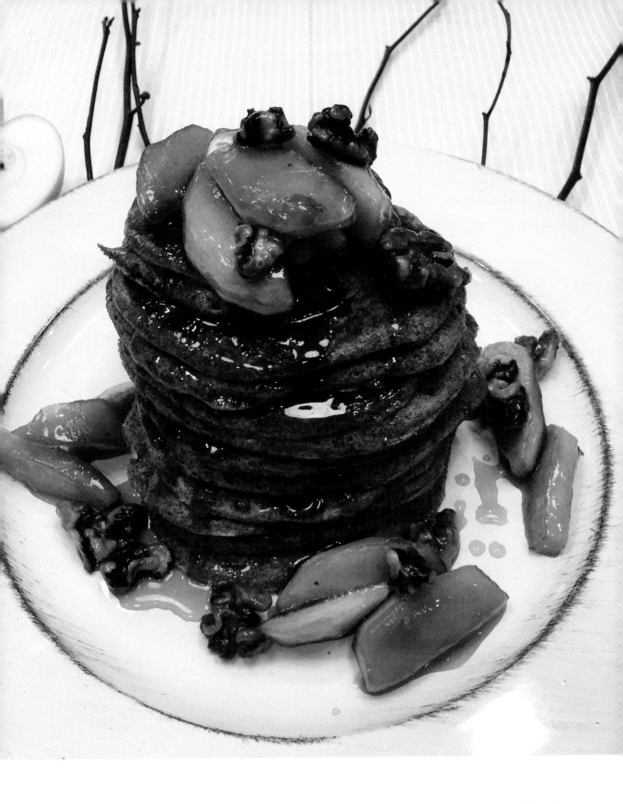

Toasted Walnut and Quinoa Pancakes with Berry Compote

For Pancakes

2 cups white, whole-wheat, flour

2 teaspoons baking powder

1 1/2 teaspoons baking soda

1 teaspoon salt

2 eggs

1 1/2 teaspoons bourbon vanilla extract

2 1/2 cups buttermilk

4 tablespoons unsalted butter, melted

3 teaspoons maple syrup

3/4 cup toasted walnuts, chopped

1 cup cooked heirloom quinoa

For Berry Compote

3 cups fresh blueberries

2/3 cup pure maple syrup

3 tablespoons water

1 tablespoon lemon zest

1/4 teaspoon ground cinnamon

1/2 teaspoon bourbon vanilla extract

Berry Compote

1. Combine two cups blueberries, maple syrup, water and cinnamon in a medium saucepan set over medium heat.

2. Simmer compote, stirring occasionally to prevent sticking for 10 minutes.

3. Reduce heat to medium low. Add the remainder of the blueberries and lemon zest, and stir frequently until compote thickens.

4. Serve warm.

Pancakes

1. Combine all dry ingredients in a medium bowl and mix well.

2. In a separate bowl, combine all wet ingredients.

3. Make a well in the dry ingredients, and pour in the liquid ingredients.

4. Sprinkle the quinoa and 1/2 cup of the walnuts into the bowl, and mix just until blended, being careful not to over mix.

5. Pour 1/4 cup of the pancake batter onto a hot, lightly oiled griddle.

6. Cook for one to two minutes then flip pancakes once air bubbles begin to rise to the surface.

7. Plate while hot, and garnish with remaining walnuts and berry compote.

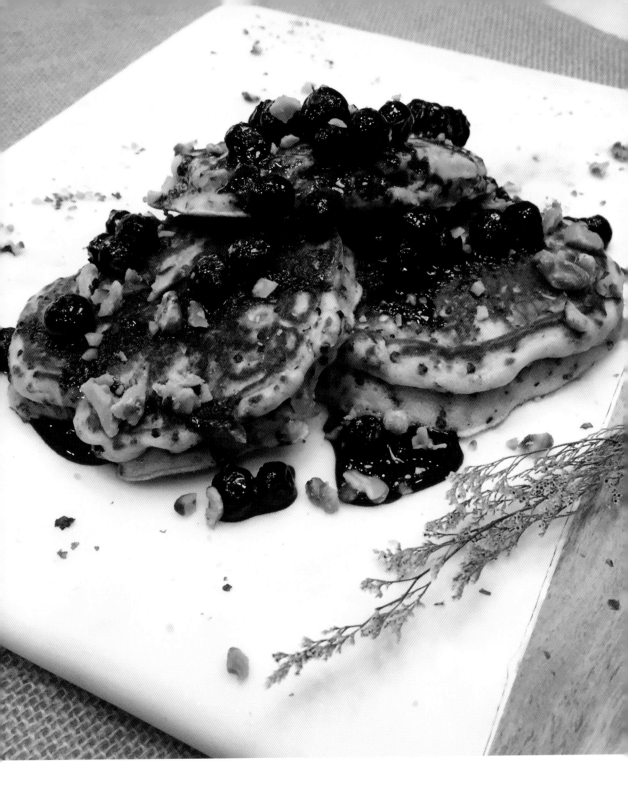

Chocolate Smoothie Bowl

2/3 cup unsweetened,
   vanilla almond milk

1/2 Hass avocado

2 frozen bananas

3 tablespoons cacao powder
   (I tend to prefer cacao powder to
   cocoa powder because it's much less
   processed.)

4 dates, seeded

1 teaspoon maple syrup

1/4 cup raspberries

1. Add all ingredients to a blender, and blend until creamy and smooth. Add more almond milk to thin it out, if necessary.

2. Adjust seasonings.

3. Serve with your favorite toppings: raspberries, bananas, chocolate goji berries, pecans, toasted coconut. The choices are endless. Have fun mixing it up!

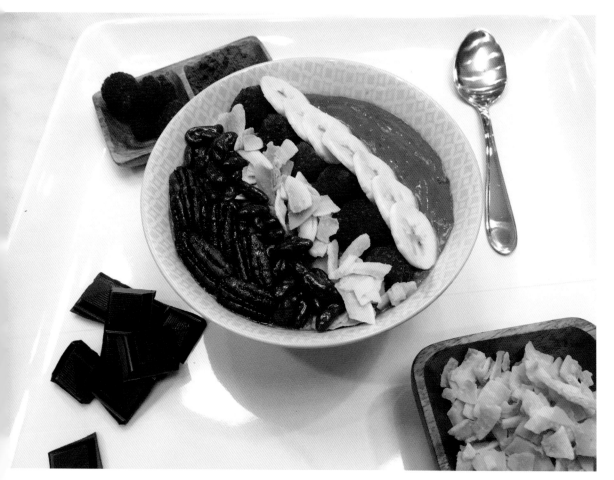

Green Smoothie Bowl

½ ripe Haas avocado

2 bananas, sliced and frozen

1 cup fresh strawberries

1 cup kale, large stems removed

1 teaspoon maple syrup

1 ½ to 2 cups unsweetened, vanilla almond milk (if berries are frozen, you'll need more liquid)

1 teaspoon maca powder

1. Add all ingredients to a blender, and blend until creamy and smooth. Add more almond milk to thin it out, if necessary.

2. Adjust seasonings.

3. Serve with your favorite toppings: strawberries, blueberries, chocolate hemp seeds or nuts. There are endless possibilities.

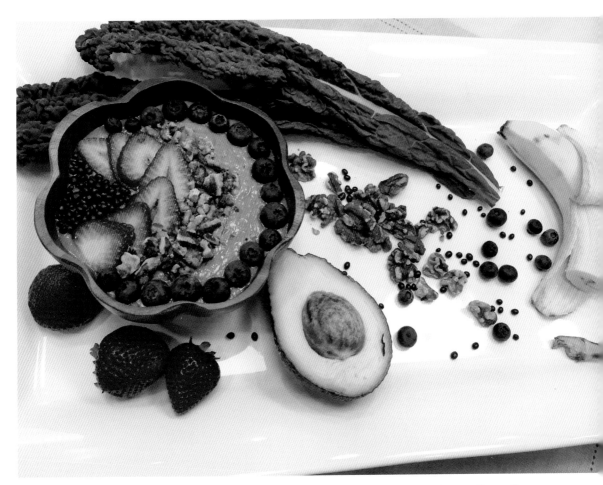

Oatmeal Blueberry Muffins

1 ¼ cups of uncooked, whole-wheat old-fashioned oatmeal

½ cup ground flax seeds

½ cup whole-wheat flower

2 tablespoons chia seeds

½ teaspoon baking soda

1 ½ teaspoons baking powder

1 teaspoon cinnamon

½ teaspoon salt

1 tablespoon lemon zest

2 tablespoons natural cinnamon applesauce

¼ cup maple syrup

⅔ cup buttermilk

½ cup Greek vanilla yogurt

2 eggs

6 tablespoons coconut oil, melted

1 ½ cups blueberries

1. Preheat your oven to 400 degrees and line your cupcake pan with reusable plastic cupcake liners (found in stores like Sur La Table or Williams Sonoma) or use cupcake liners.

2. Mix all your dry ingredients in a large mixing until well incorporated.

3. In a separate bowl, combine all wet ingredients, and mix well to incorporate.

4. Make a well in the middle of the dry ingredients.

5. Pour the wet mixture into dry ingredients, and mix to combine.

6. Fold in blueberries just until incorporated and spoon mixture into muffin pan. If you over mix, your muffins won't be airy and light. Top muffins with remaining blueberries.

7. Bake until tops are slightly golden.

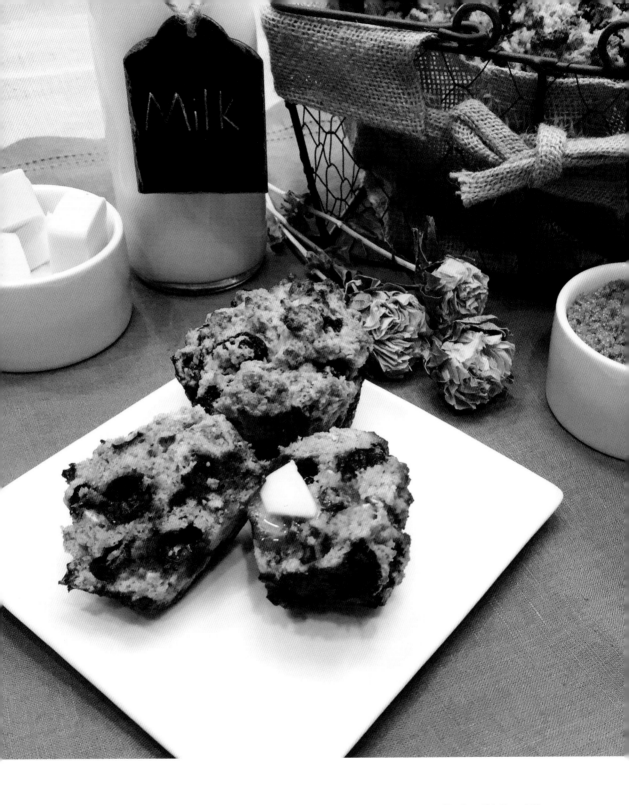

Blueberry Oatmeal with Granny Smith Apples and Candied Pecans

1 cup whole-wheat, old-fashioned oats

¼ cup chia seeds

3 cups unsweetened, vanilla almond milk

1 ½ teaspoons bourbon vanilla extract

1 teaspoon salt

1 teaspoon cinnamon

½ teaspoon nutmeg

1 Granny Smith apple, sliced

2 cups blueberries

2 tablespoons maple syrup

½ cup candied pecans (Hint: You can buy these already made. I won't tell, if you don't.)

1. Combine oats, chia seeds, almond milk, vanilla, salt, cinnamon, nutmeg, apples, 1 ½ cups blueberries and maple syrup in a medium saucepan over medium-high heat.

2. Bring oatmeal to a boil then reduce heat to medium and let simmer while constantly stirring until oatmeal thickens. The chia seeds are heavier than the oat flakes, and constantly stirring prevents the seeds from sinking to the bottom of the pot and creating lumps or burning.

3. Adjust seasoning, and garnish with candied pecans and fresh blueberries.

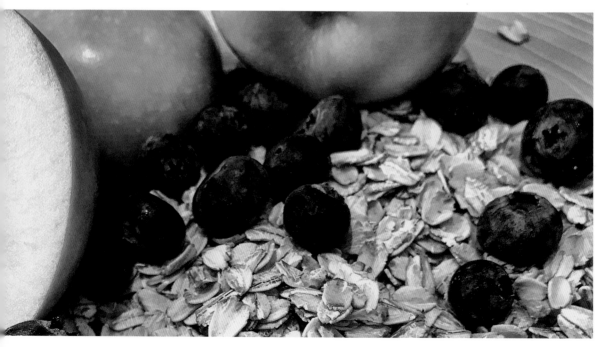

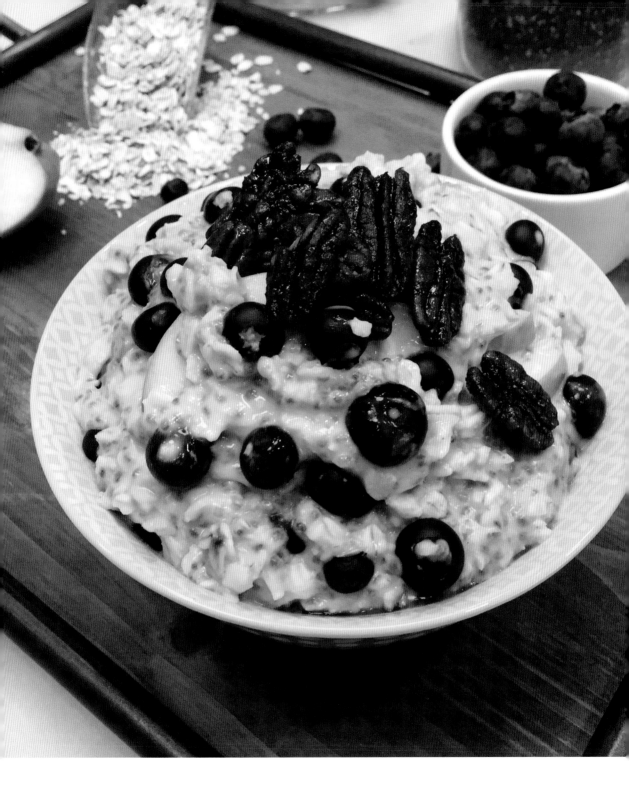

German Chocolate Cake Oatmeal

For Oatmeal

1 cup whole-grain, old-fashioned oats

3 cups unsweetened, vanilla coconut milk

2 tablespoons cacao powder (the purest form of chocolate you can consume)

1 cup unsweetened coconut

2 tablespoons maple syrup

2 tablespoons ground flaxseed

1 teaspoon bourbon vanilla extract

1 teaspoon salt

¼ cup shaved chocolate

½ cup toasted pecans, chopped

For Caramel Pecan Topping

10 dates, pitted and chopped

¼ cup sweet potato puree (I took a small sweet potato and roasted it at 375 degrees for about 40 minutes, or until it was soft. This produces a sweeter potato because the sugars of the potato caramelize.)

2 tablespoons applesauce

2-3 tablespoons hot apple juice

6 tablespoons shredded coconut

2 tablespoons toasted pecans, chopped

Caramel Topping

1. Combine the chopped dates, sweet potato puree, applesauce, hot apple juice and four tablespoons of shredded coconut in a small bowl. Let sit until the dates have softened a little. This helps with the processing.

2. Pour the sweet potato mixture into the bowl of a food processor, and process until smooth.

3. Fold in coconut and pecans.

Oatmeal

1. Combine oats, coconut milk, powder, ½ cup coconut, maple syrup, flaxseed, vanilla and salt in a medium saucepan over medium-high heat.

2. Bring mixture to a simmer, stirring often to prevent sticking.

3. Your oatmeal is done once it's creamy and fluffy. If it's not as loose as you'd like it to be, just add more coconut milk until you reach the desired consistency.

4. Adjust your seasonings, remove from heat and garnish with caramel pecan topping, toasted pecans and shaved chocolate.

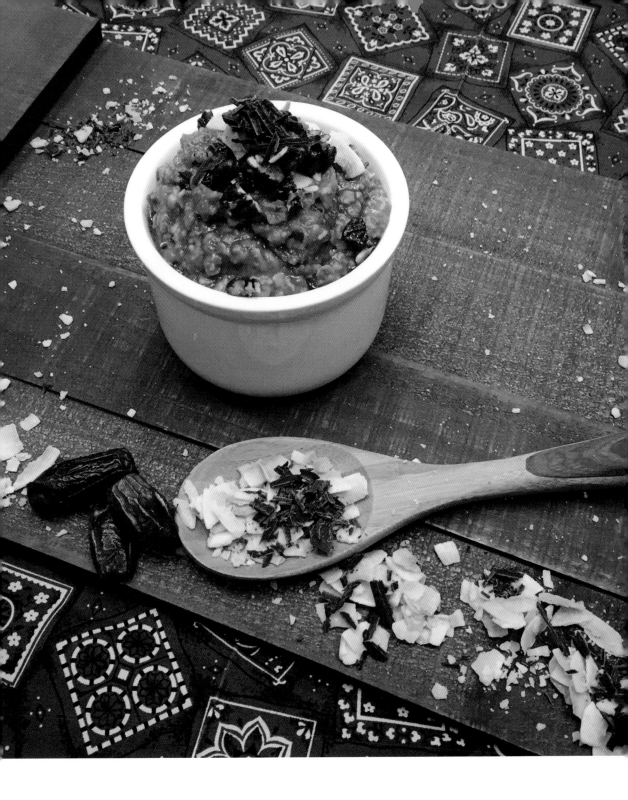

Peanut Butter and Banana Oatmeal with Peanut Granola

For oatmeal

- 1 cup whole-grain, old-fashioned oats
- 3 cups unsweetened, vanilla almond milk
- 2 tablespoons creamy peanut butter (if you like peanut butter like I do, then add more)
- 1 1/2 teaspoons cinnamon
- 1/2 teaspoon salt
- 1 tablespoon maple syrup
- 1 1/2 bananas, chopped

For Peanut Granola

- 1/2 cup chunky peanut butter (creamy peanut butter works just as well)
- 1/2 cup pure maple syrup
- 1/4 cup coconut oil
- 1/2 teaspoon salt
- 3 cups whole-grain, old-fashioned oats
- 1 cup roasted peanuts

Peanut Granola

1. Preheat your oven to 300 degrees.
2. In a bowl, combine the peanut butter, maple syrup, oil and salt.
3. Fold in your oats and peanuts.
4. Pour your granola onto a large baking sheet.
5. Bake for about 30 minutes. Half way through the baking process, toss the granola with a spatula or spoon to ensure even baking.
6. Remove from the oven, and let cool before using.

Oatmeal

1. Combine oats, almond milk, peanut butter, one banana, cinnamon, salt and maple syrup in a medium saucepan over medium-high heat.
2. Bring mixture to a simmer, stirring often to prevent sticking.
3. Your oatmeal is done once it's creamy and fluffy. If it's not as loose as you'd like it to be, add more almond milk until you reach the desired consistency.
4. Adjust your seasonings, and remove from heat.
5. Garnish with remaining chopped bananas and peanut granola.

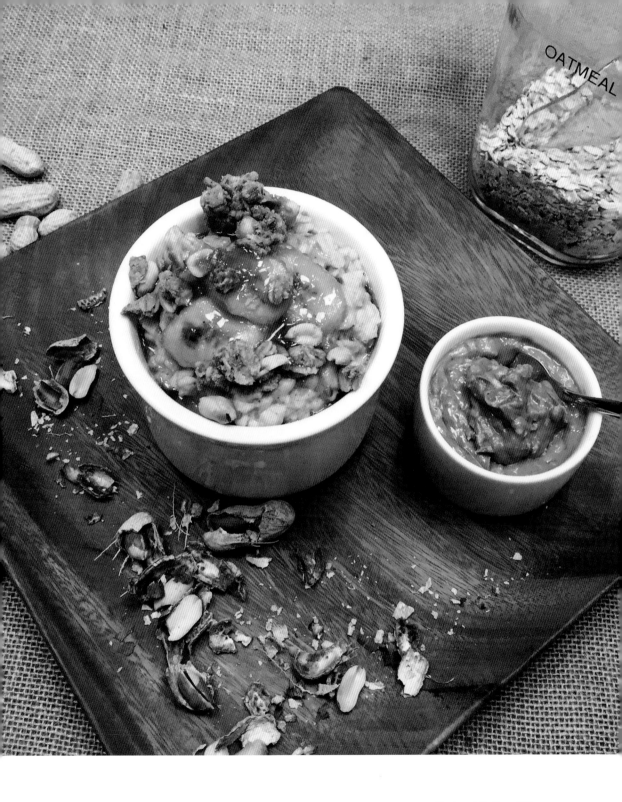

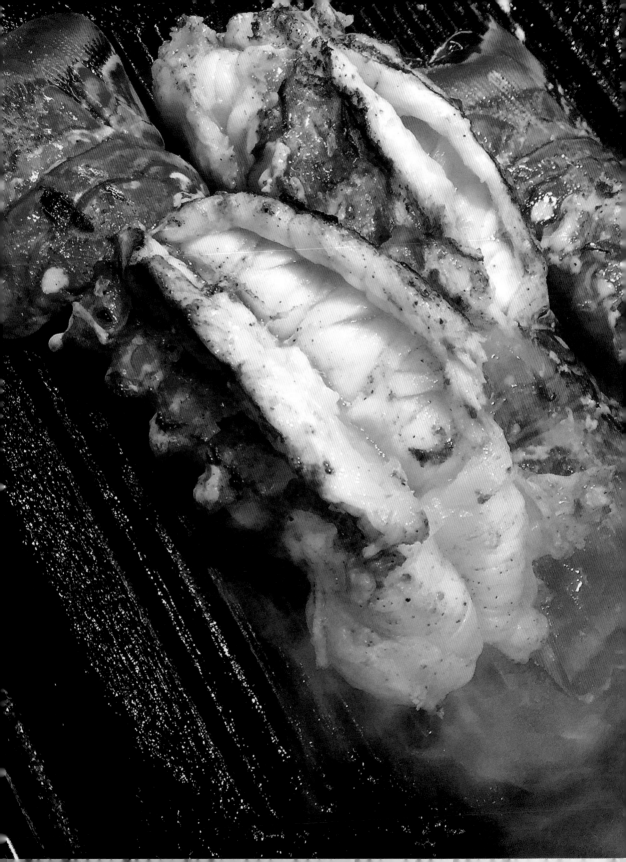

Let's do lunch!

Just as breakfast kickstarts a productive day, lunch is that meal that keeps you going. We often find ourselves working through lunch and then stuff ourselves at dinner to compensate for the meal we missed.

By eating a balanced lunch, you're providing your mind and body the fuel to finish the day just as strongly as it began.

Eating Lunch to Win

Avoid eating fast food like burgers and chips for lunch. Fatty foods take longer to digest, making you feel lethargic and hampering your productivity.

Twice Baked Seafood Spaghetti Squash

For Squash

- 2 medium spaghetti squash
- 2 tablespoons extra virgin olive oil
- 1 tablespoon dry Italian herbs
- ½ small onion, diced
- 3 cloves garlic, sliced
- 2 cups fire-roasted tomato sauce
- ½ pound medium shrimp, peeled deveined
- 2 medium lobster tails, split, deveined, shell removed except tail fin
- 1 medium zucchini, cut in half, then sliced
- 1 cup white, sharp cheddar
- ½ cup asiago cheese
- salt and pepper

For Tomato Sauce

- 2 tablespoons olive oil
- 1 cup onions, chopped
- 2 teaspoons salt
- ¼ teaspoon pepper
- 3 garlic cloves, sliced thin
- 1 tablespoon fresh thyme
- 3 ½ cups canned, fire-roasted tomatoes

Squash

1. Preheat your oven to 400 degrees.

2. Slice two spaghetti squash in half lengthwise, and scoop out seeds and stringy flesh.

3. Place squash on a foiled, lined baking sheet and drizzle with one of the tablespoons of oil, and season with salt, pepper and dry Italian herbs.

4. Turn squash cut side down on baking sheet and bake for 40 minutes, or until soft.

5. In a large sauté pan over medium heat, sauté the onion and garlic in the remaining olive oil, and stir often until the onion is translucent.

6. Add in the zucchini, and continue to stir until it's softened.

7. Add tomato sauce to the zucchini/ onion mixture.

8. Once the sauce is hot, add in the shrimp and lobster, lower the heat and let simmer until the lobster and shrimp are just starting to turn opaque.

9. Adjust seasonings, and remove your pan from the heat. Let it sit until squash is ready.

10. Remove the squash from oven, and use a fork to gently pull the squash flesh in the same direction as the strands to achieve the longest pieces of "spaghetti."

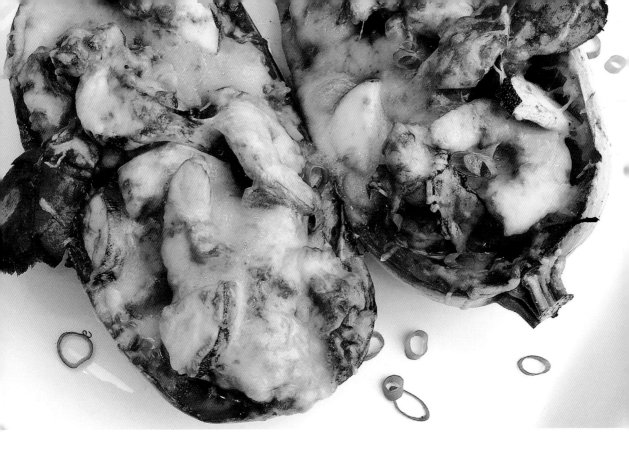

11. Fold the squash into the seafood mixture along with ¼ cup of the white cheddar and Asiago cheeses then place back into the hulls.

12. Sprinkle each squash with the remaining cheese.

13. Place the stuffed squash back in the oven, and bake until the cheese starts to bubble.

Tomato Sauce

1. Sauté onions in a medium pan over medium heat.

2. Season with salt and pepper, and stir often until onions are soft.

3. Add garlic, and cook until softened, being careful not to let the mixture burn.

4. Add thyme.

5. Stir in roasted tomatoes with juices and bring to a boil.

6. Reduce heat and bring to a simmer, stirring often to prevent sticking, until sauce has thickened.

7. Purée sauce in a food processor.

8. Adjust seasonings, and let sauce cool.

Curry Sweet Potato Leek Soup

2 medium leeks, chopped and cleaned
(use the white parts only)

1 Bosc pear, peeled, cored and sliced

1 medium sweet potato, cut into cubes

2 tablespoons coconut oil

½ tablespoon plus 1 teaspoon curry
powder (adjust to your liking)

Kosher salt and freshly ground pepper

3 cups vegetable broth

1 bay leaf

½ cup unsweetened coconut milk

1 teaspoon olive oil

1. Melt coconut oil in a medium saucepan over medium-high heat.

2. Add in curry powder. You should smell the curry throughout your kitchen as it starts to heat up.

3. Add the pears and leeks, and season with salt and pepper. Stir frequently until the pears and leeks have softened.

4. Add the vegetable broth, and bring to a boil.

5. Reduce the heat to medium, and add the sweet potatoes.

6. As the soup simmers, add in the bay leaf and allow the soup to cook until the sweet potatoes are soft.

7. Remove the bay leaf, and pour the soup into a blender in batches, if necessary.

8. Blend soup until smooth.

9. Pour the soup back into the saucepan, and whisk in coconut milk.

10. Let simmer for about 10 minutes. If soup is too thick for your taste, add a little more broth.

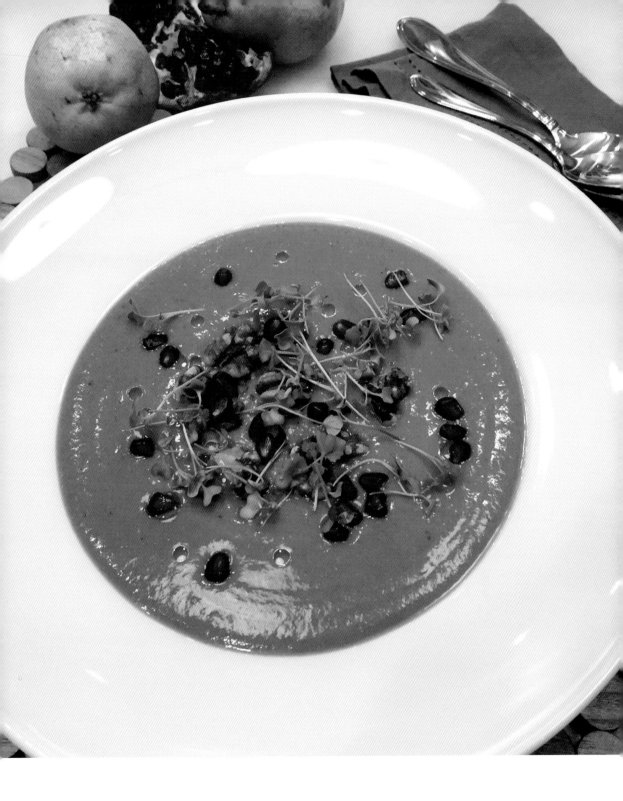

Roasted Portobello Butter Lettuce "Tacos" with Pineapple Corn Relish

For Tacos

3 large portobello caps, stems removed, sliced into strips

1 tablespoon olive oil

Kosher salt and freshly ground pepper

1 ½ teaspoons cumin

½ teaspoon smoked paprika

1 ½ tablespoons balsamic vinegar

4-6 medium butter lettuce leaves, washed and patted dry

½ cup chopped fresh cilantro leaves

Sriracha sauce

For Pineapple Corn Relish

1 ½ cups whole-kernel corn

1 ½ cups fresh pineapple, diced

⅓ cup finely diced red onion

¼ cup chopped, fresh cilantro leaves

1 jalapeño, seeded and diced

½ teaspoon ground cumin

Kosher salt

2 tablespoons fresh pineapple juice

1 tablespoon fresh lime juice

Tacos

1. Preheat your oven to 400 degrees.

2. Combine mushrooms and olive oil in a medium mixing bowl, and toss.

3. On a foiled, parchment-lined baking sheet, lay the mushrooms out evenly.

4. Season evenly with salt, pepper, cumin and paprika.

5. Drizzle balsamic over seasoned mushroom slices.

6. Roast until the mushrooms are cooked through and soft.

7. Remove from the oven and reserve until ready for use.

8. Line the center of each butter lettuce leaf with three to four pieces of roasted mushrooms.

Pineapple Corn Relish:

1. Combine all ingredients in a medium bowl.

2. Fold together until well incorporated.

3. Adjust seasoning, and reserve until ready for use.

4. Place on top of each taco with fresh cilantro and Sriracha.

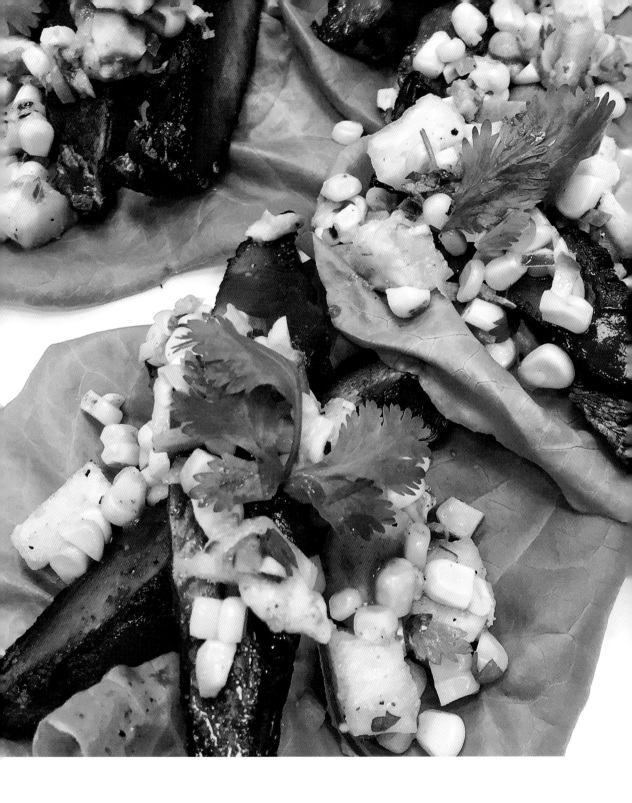

Romaine Turkey "Tacos" with Avocado Cilantro Salad

For Turkey Tacos

1 tablespoon olive oil

1 small red onion, chopped

3 cloves garlic, minced

1 pound lean ground turkey

kosher salt and freshly ground
    black pepper

1 teaspoon smoked paprika

1 ½ teaspoons red pepper flakes

2 teaspoons ground cumin

2 teaspoons chili powder

¾ cup low-sodium chicken broth

12 Romaine lettuce leaves, doubled up,
    for serving

For Avocado Cilantro Salad

3 Hass avocados, diced

2 cups cherry tomatoes

½ medium red onion, sliced

2 garlic cloves, minced

¼ cup cilantro, chopped

2 tablespoons olive oil

3 tablespoons fresh lime juice

2 teaspoons honey

1 tablespoon Tequila (ah yes, you read
    that correctly)

Kosher salt and fresh ground pepper

2 teaspoons cumin

1 teaspoon chili powder

Tacos

1. Sautée onions in olive oil in a medium skillet over medium-high heat until soft.

2. Combine turkey and garlic with onions.

3. Season with salt, pepper, paprika, red pepper flakes, cumin and chili powder.

4. Cook while breaking up turkey until it's cooked through and resembles crumbles.

5. Add chicken broth, and simmer until liquid has reduced.

6. Adjust seasonings.

7. Line the center of each Romaine lettuce leaf with turkey mixture.

Avocado Cilantro Salad

1. Combine avocado, tomatoes, onions, garlic and cilantro in a large salad bowl.

2. In a small bowl, combine remaining ingredients, and whisk vigorously to incorporate flavors.

3. Adjust seasonings, and use to top each lettuce taco.

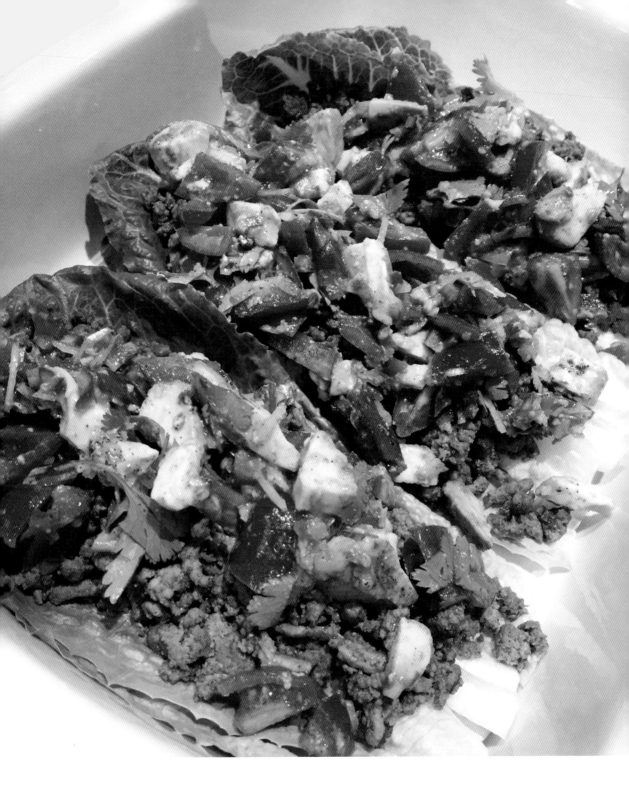

Black Lentil and Kale Soup with Turkey Andouille Sausage

1 tablespoon grape seed oil

½ cup turkey andouille sausage, sliced

1 medium onion, chopped

2 celery ribs, chopped

2 carrots, chopped

3 cloves garlic, sliced

Kosher salt and fresh ground
   black pepper

1 ½ cups beluga lentils, rinsed

4 cups low-sodium chicken broth

1 bay leaf

1 tablespoon fresh thyme leaves

½ bunch kale, stemmed, rinsed,
   chopped (about 3 cups)

Sour cream

1. Brown sausages in oil over medium-high heat in a large saucepot.

2. Remove sausages from pot, and reserve.

3. Discard all but one tablespoon of oil left in the saucepot.

4. Add onion, celery, carrots, and garlic and sauté, stirring until they start to soften.

5. Season with salt and pepper.

6. Stir in lentils, making sure they get coated all over with the flavor of the aromatics.

7. Add in broth, cover and bring to a boil.

8. Reduce heat to medium, add in thyme and bay leaf.

9. Simmer partially covered, until lentils are tender.

10. Stir in kale, leave partially covered until kale wilts.

11. Return sausage to the soup, and cook just until sausage is warmed through.

12. Remove bay leaf, and adjust seasonings.

13. Ladle soup in a bowl, and top with sour cream.

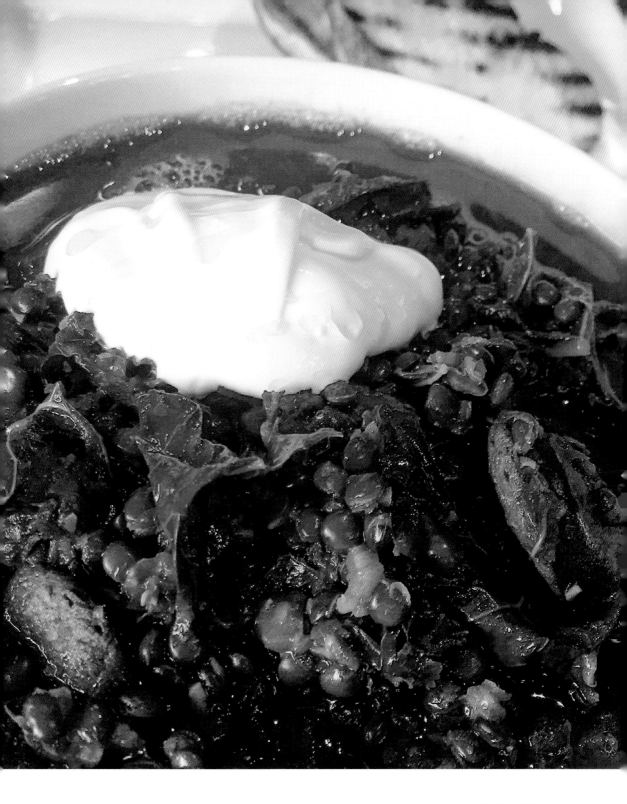

Lentil Penne Pasta with Turkey Meat Sauce

1 tablespoon olive oil

½ cup turkey kielbasa

1 pound ground turkey

1 medium red onion, chopped

4 garlic cloves, minced

2 teaspoons dried Italian seasoning

2 teaspoons smoked paprika

1 teaspoon Creole seasoning

3 cups tomato sauce (recipe found in
the Twice Baked Seafood Spaghetti
Squash p. 52)

2 cups lentil penne pasta, cooked

Asiago cheese, shaved

Kosher salt and freshly ground pepper

1. Brown turkey sausage in one tablespoon of the oil in a large sauté pan over medium-high heat.

2. Remove from the pan, and reserve until ready for use.

3. Pour off all but one tablespoon of the oil left in the pan, and add the ground turkey. Cook until brown and turkey is broken up to resemble crumbles.

4. Reduce the heat to medium and add onion, garlic, Italian seasonings, paprika, and Creole seasoning until onion is tender.

5. Add tomato sauce, and reduce the heat to medium low.

6. Simmer until sauce thickens then incorporate sausages into the sauce until sausages are warmed through.

7. Adjust seasonings, and toss pasta with meat sauce

8. Serve topped with shaved asiago cheese in large bowl.

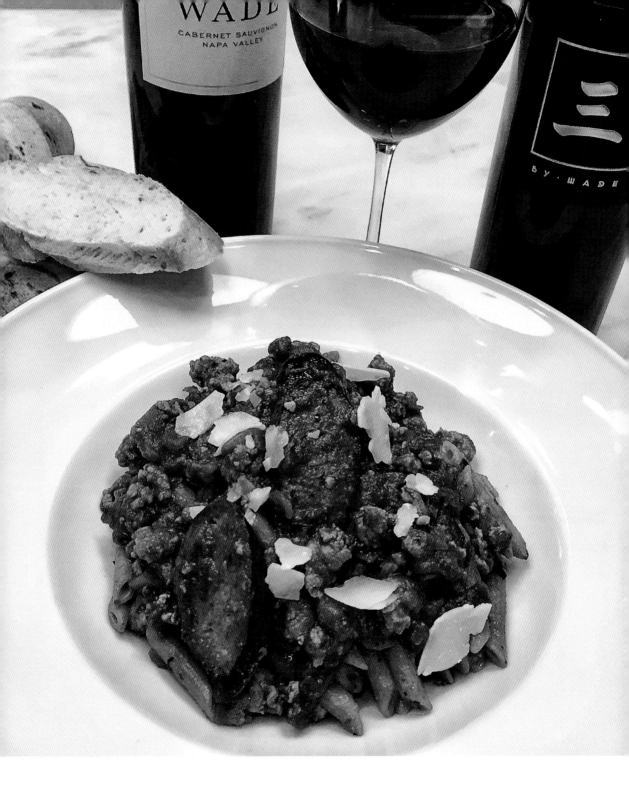

Grilled Red Snapper with Citrus Avocado Vinaigrette

For Snapper

Four 6-ounce snapper filets

Salt and fresh ground pepper

For avocado vinaigrette

1 Hass avocado peeled, seeded and diced

2 oranges supremed (a fancy word for sectioned, use it to impress your friends)

2 teaspoons shallots, minced

1 garlic clove, minced

2 roma tomatoes, seeded and diced

1 teaspoon jalapeño pepper, minced

2 tablespoons fresh cilantro, chopped

½ cup grape seed oil

¼ cup rice wine vinegar

3 tablespoons fresh lime juice

3 tablespoons fresh orange juice

¼ teaspoon finely grated lime zest

¼ teaspoon orange zest

1 tablespoon honey

Kosher salt and freshly ground pepper

How to supreme an orange:

1. Cut off the top, so that the orange flesh is visible.

2. Do the same thing on the bottom, so that the flesh is visible and the orange sits flat.

3. Cut from top to bottom curving the knife to the shape of the orange.

4. Repeat this step all the way around until all the peel is removed.

5. Cut in between the white sections, placing your knife as close to the white membrane as possible, and slice at a slight angle to the core. If done correctly, you'll be left with skinless orange wedges.

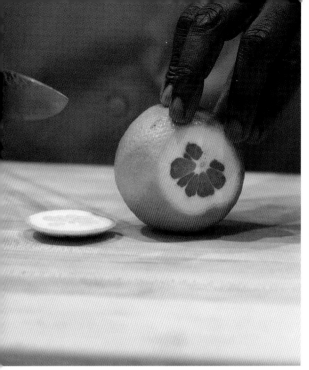
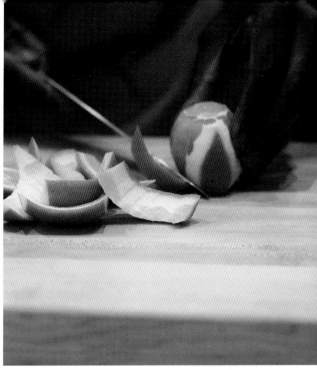
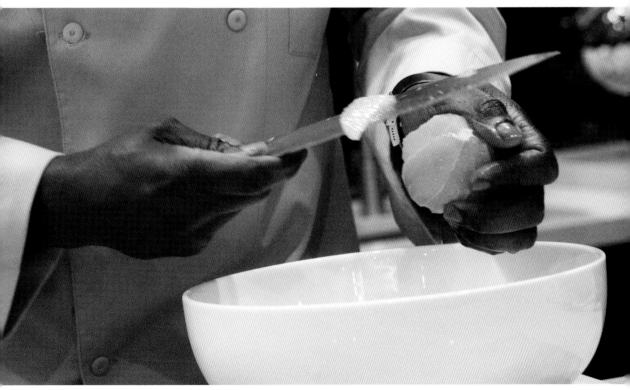

Snapper

1. Season snapper on both sides with salt and pepper.

2. Place snapper on a heated, oiled grill rack.

3. Grill five minutes on each side, or until the fish flakes easily when tested with a fork. Start with the skin side down. You'll be tempted to look to see if it's ready, but fight this urge. It's a sure fire way to mess up the skin and your final presentation. When it's ready, the fish will turn easily.

4. Remove, and reserve until ready.

Avocado Vinaigrette

1. In a medium bowl, combine avocado, segmented oranges, shallots, garlic, tomatoes, pepper and cilantro.

2. In a separate bowl, combine vinegar, lime juice, orange juice, zest and honey.

3. Vigorously whisk in oil and season to taste.

4. Whisk wet mixture into the solid ingredients, and adjust seasonings, if necessary.

5. Use mixture to top snapper, which should be served skin side up.

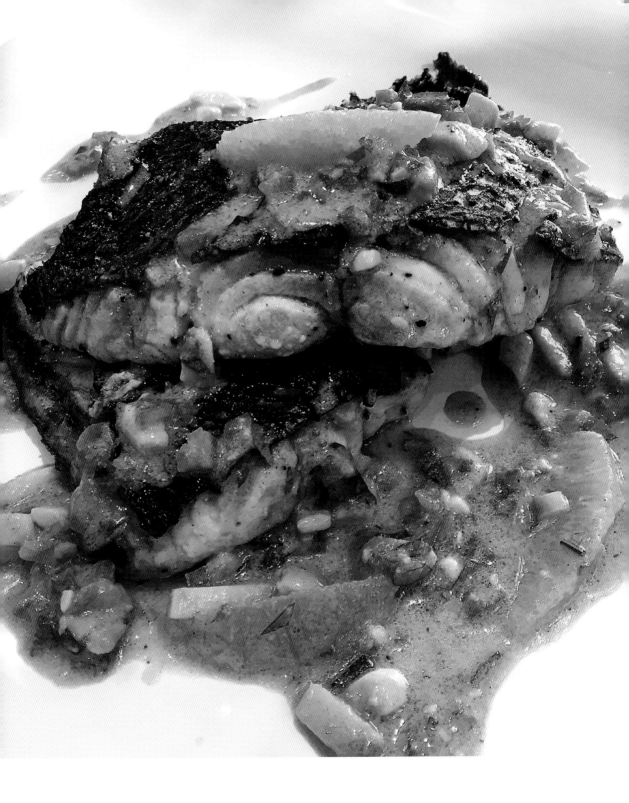

Asian Vegetable and Noodle Soup

1 tablespoon vegetable oil

1 small onion, sliced thin

2 cloves garlic, chopped

2 small carrots, peeled and sliced into
small rounds

2 teaspoons finely grated, peeled ginger

1 red bell pepper cored, seeded
and sliced

1 teaspoon crushed red pepper flakes

4 cups low-sodium vegetable broth

4 cups rainbow Swiss chard, torn

2 tablespoons ponzu sauce

1 teaspoon fish sauce

Kosher salt and fresh ground
black pepper

1 package wide rice noodles, cooked

2 boiled eggs

Sambal

Cilantro

1. Add oil to a large pot, and cook onions, garlic, carrots, ginger, and pepper over medium heat stirring until vegetables are just beginning to soften.

2. Add red pepper flakes, and cook for one minute more.

3. Add broth, and bring to a boil.

4. Reduce heat and add ponzu and fish sauce.

5. Let soup simmer until flavors fully incorporate.

6. Add greens, and stir occasionally until they are tender.

7. Season with salt and pepper.

8. Divide noodles among bowls, and ladle soup over them.

9. Garnish with half of a boiled egg, cilantro and sambal.

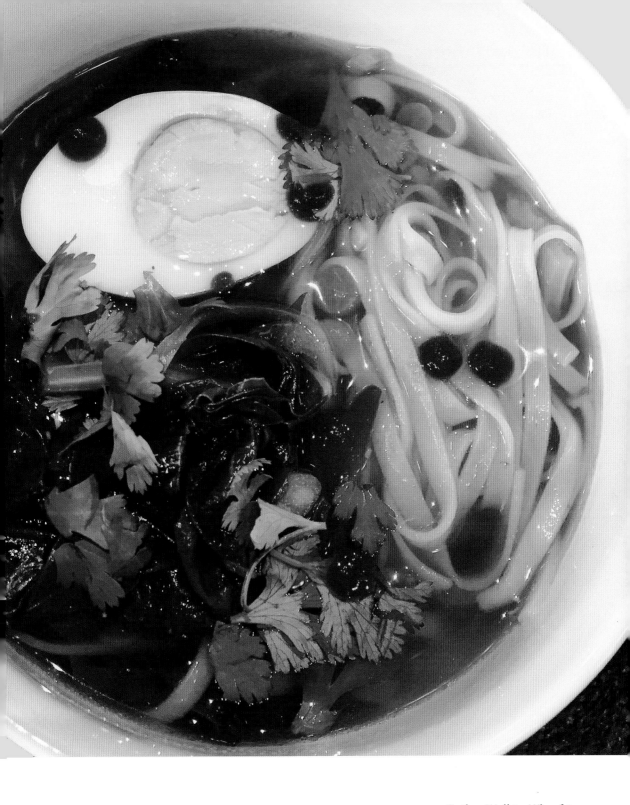

Lobster Masala

3 tablespoons grape seed oil

4 medium lobster tails, deveined, shell removed except tail fin

½ tablespoon curry powder

½ teaspoon five-spice powder

1 cup onions

1 green bell pepper, chopped

1 red chili pepper, seeded and chopped

2 curry leaves

1 bay leaf

1 ½ tablespoons ginger-garlic paste (You can easily make your own with 1 cup ginger chopped, 1 cup garlic cloves, 1 teaspoon turmeric powder, 1 teaspoon curry powder and 1 tablespoon canola oil. Then use a food processor to create a smooth paste.)

½ cup fresh cilantro, chopped

1 tablespoon toasted coriander seeds, crushed

1 teaspoon toasted cumin seeds, crushed

1 teaspoon red chili powder

1 ½ teaspoons garam masala powder

½ teaspoon turmeric powder

1 ½ cups fire-roasted, chopped tomatoes

½ cup vegetable broth

2 pounds fresh okra

Salt and fresh ground black pepper

1. Season lobster tails with curry powder, five spice, and salt and pepper.

2. Brown lobster tails in two tablespoons of the oil in a saucepan over medium-high heat.

3. Remove lobster tails from the pan and reserve until ready for use.

4. In the same pan, cook onions and ginger-garlic paste until onions become soft.

5. Add bell pepper, red chili, curry leaves, bay leaf, coriander, cumin, chili powder, garam masala and turmeric.

6. Cook until fragrant.

7. Add in tomatoes, and season with salt and pepper.

8. Stir until tomatoes start to break down.

9. Add a little salt so that tomatoes will cook fast.

10. Once the tomatoes soften, add in the broth, reduce heat and let simmer.

11. Heat a separate medium pan with the remaining one tablespoon of oil and brown the okra, but don't let it get too soft.

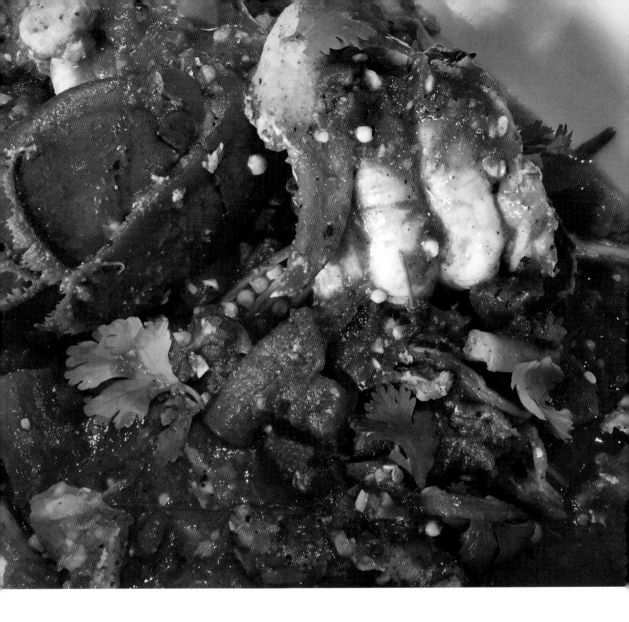

12. Add the fried okra to simmering tomato sauce, increase heat to medium high and let it come to a boil.

13. Add chopped cilantro, and stir to fully incorporate. If your sauce gets too thick, use more vegetable broth to thin it out.

14. Reduce heat to medium, add reserved lobster tails and cover pan.

15. Cook for five to seven minutes.

Conch Salad

4 pieces fresh conch, tenderized and diced (If you don't have a tenderizer at home, you can ask the fishmonger at the market to do it for you. I like to have mine run through the machine twice to make sure it's extra tender.)

2 stalks celery, minced

1 habanero pepper, minced

3 limes, juiced

2 oranges, segmented

2 oranges, juiced

1 red bell pepper, minced

¼ cup red onion, minced

2 teaspoons kosher salt

1 tablespoon agave nectar

1. Combine all ingredients in a medium bowl and adjust seasonings.

2. Cover and refrigerate for 20 minutes.

3. Remove from the refrigerator, and serve.

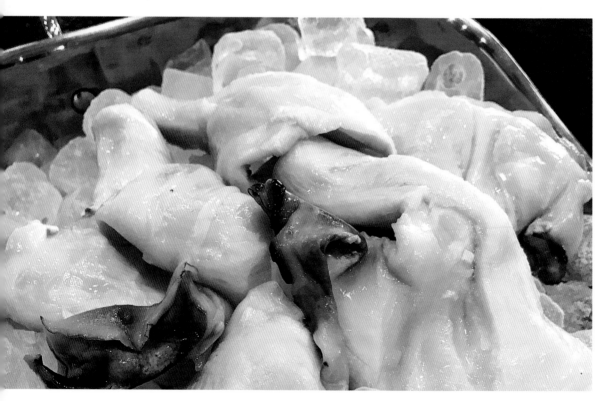

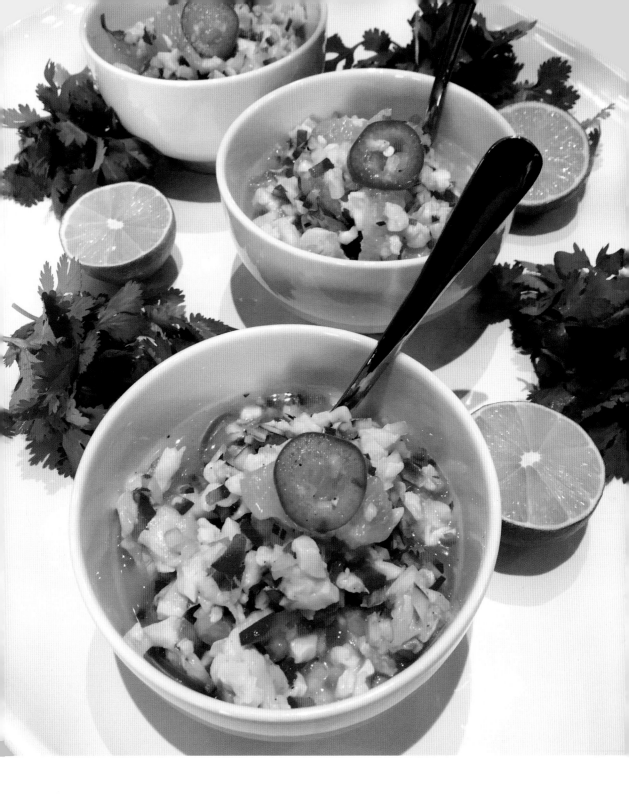

Stewed Conch

6 medium size conch, cleaned and
    tenderized
3 strips bacon, chopped
½ cup white whole-wheat flour
1 small onion, finely chopped
1 can fire-roasted tomatoes
1 teaspoon red pepper flakes
1 tablespoon fresh thyme
2 bay leaves
4 cups low-sodium, vegetable broth
2 medium sweet potatoes, peeled, cut
    into medium dice
Juice of 1 lime
Kosher salt and pepper to taste

1. Place conch in a large saucepan, cover with water and parboil uncovered until tender. Watch water closely because it's almost guaranteed to boil over if you don't. (It's happened to me more than once.)

2. Render fat from bacon in a medium pan over medium heat.

3. Using a slotted spoon, remove bacon and reserve until ready for use.

4. Add flour to the bacon drippings, and stir until golden brown.

5. Add onion, roasted tomatoes, red pepper flakes, thyme and bay leaves.

6. Whisk in three cups of broth into the flour mixture, and simmer stirring occasionally until sauce thickens slightly. If sauce is too thick, feel free to thin it out with added broth.

7. Add conch to the sauce along with sweet potatoes, and cover.

8. Simmer until conch and potatoes are fork tender.

9. Finish with fresh lime juice, and adjust seasonings.

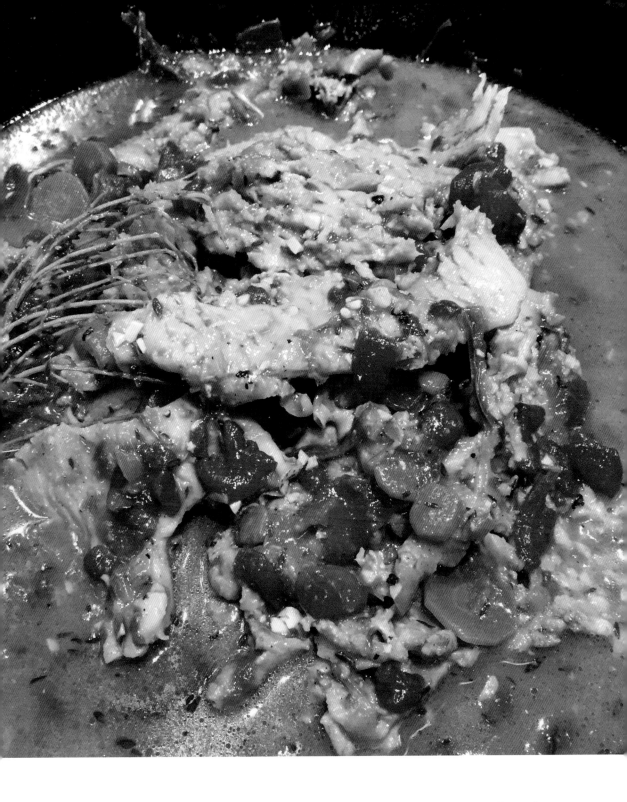

Asian Watermelon Blueberry Salad

4 cups watermelon, seeded and cubed

1 pint fresh blueberries

2 tablespoons fresh lime juice

2 tablespoons fresh orange juice

1 teaspoon freshly grated ginger

1 tablespoon rice wine vinegar

2 teaspoons ponzu

1 tablespoon fish sauce

2 teaspoons honey

1 teaspoon Sriracha

2 tablespoons fresh mint, chopped

¼ cup fresh cilantro, chopped

Kosher salt and pepper to taste

1. Combine watermelon and blueberries in a large bowl.

2. In a separate bowl, whisk together lime juice, orange juice, ginger, rice wine vinegar, ponzu, fish sauce, honey and Sriracha.

3. Season with salt and pepper.

4. Pour dressing over the watermelon and blueberries.

5. Fold in the mint and cilantro.

6. Adjust seasonings and serve.

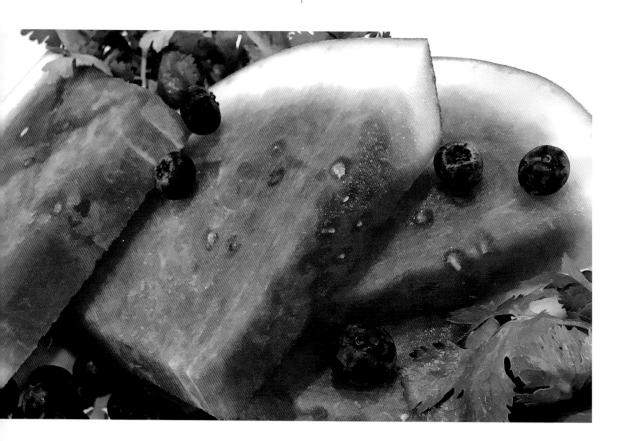

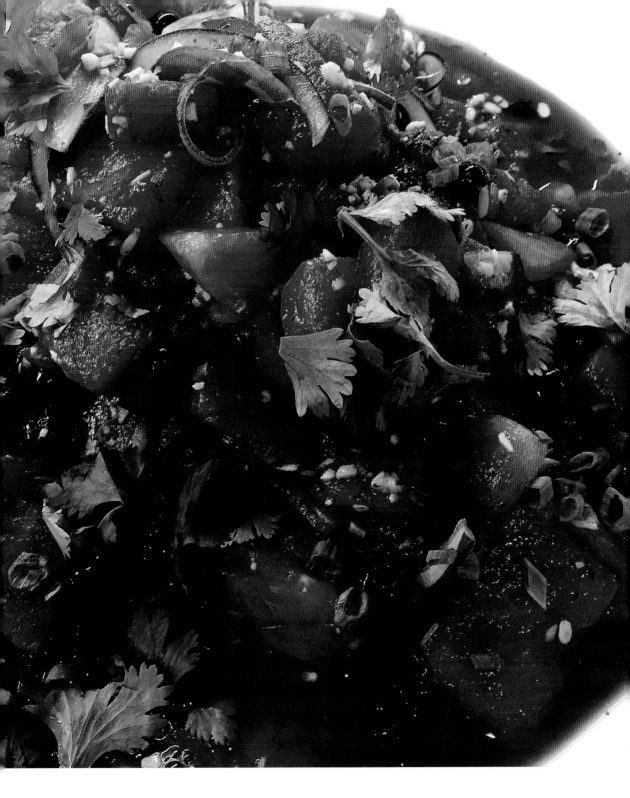

Chicken Chili with Smoked Chicken Sausage

2 tablespoons canola oil

1 pound smoked chicken sausage, sliced into ½ inch pieces

1 ½ pounds ground chicken thigh meat

1 ½ cups red onions, chopped

4 cloves garlic, sliced

1 red bell pepper, cored and chopped

½ cup celery

2 tablespoons chili powder

3 teaspoons ground cumin

2 teaspoons smoked paprika

2 teaspoons garlic powder

1 teaspoon onion powder

2 teaspoons red pepper flakes

3 teaspoons dried oregano

1 ½ cups beer

3 cups canned, fire-roasted tomatoes

2 tablespoons tomato paste

2 cups chicken broth

Kosher salt and fresh ground black pepper

4 cups red kidney beans, drained and rinsed

1. Brown sausage in two tablespoons of oil in a large heavy pot over medium-high heat.

2. Using a slotted spoon, remove sausage from the pot, drain on paper towels and reserve until ready for use.

3. Add the ground chicken to the pot. Cook until brown and chicken is broken up to resemble crumbles.

4. Add the onions, garlic, bell pepper, celery, spices, and sift often to incorporate flavors.

5. Add beer. Cook until the foam subsides and liquid reduces by half.

6. Add the tomatoes, tomato paste, chicken broth, and season with salt and pepper.

7. Stir well, and bring to a boil.

8. Lower the heat to medium low and simmer for 15 minutes, uncovered, stirring occasionally to prevent the chili from sticking to the bottom of the pot.

9. Add beans, and reserved sausage.

10. Stir for 10 minutes until beans and sausage are heated through.

11. Serve with your favorite toppings: avocado, red onion, cilantro, sour cream, cheese or limes.

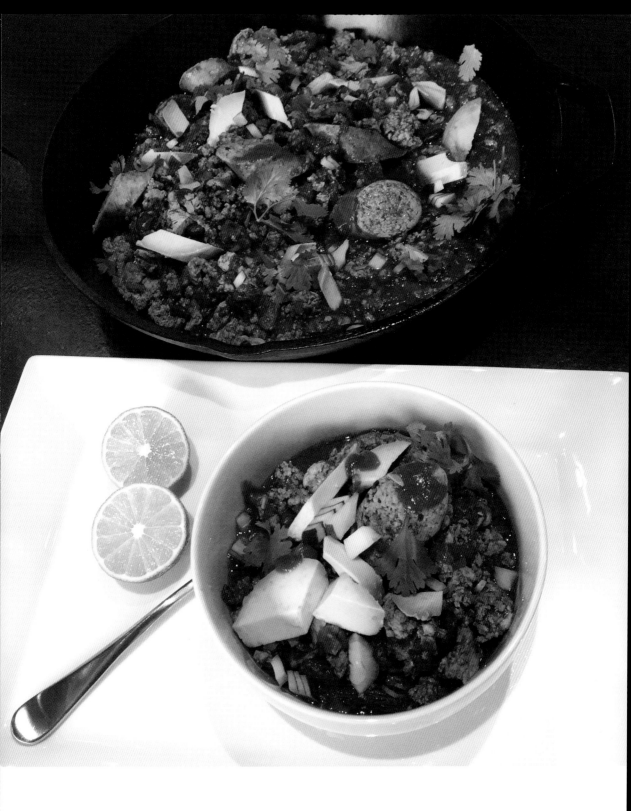

Grilled Portobello with Lobster and Shrimp Salad

For Portobello Mushrooms

6 tablespoons grape seed oil

3 tablespoons fig balsamic vinegar

3 garlic cloves, minced

1 tablespoon fresh thyme

6 large portobello mushrooms,
   stemmed with gills scraped out

Kosher salt and fresh ground pepper

For Lobster and Shrimp Salad

¼ cup rice wine vinegar

3 tablespoons whole grain mustard

1 tablespoon honey

2 tablespoons shallots, minced

1 garlic clove, minced

½ cup grape seed oil

Kosher salt and freshly ground pepper

¾ pound cooked lobster meat, chopped

½ pound medium cooked shrimp

1 ½ cups ripe mango, chopped

1 ¼ cup fresh raw corn from about
   2-3 ears

1 cup micro greens

Mushrooms

1. Heat grill to medium-high heat.

2. Whisk oil, fig balsamic vinegar, garlic and thyme in small bowl, and season with salt and pepper.

3. Arrange mushroom caps on foil-lined baking sheet, gill side up.

4. Generously spoon dressing into each mushroom.

5. Place mushrooms on grill, gill side down, and grill until edges start to soften.

6. Turn mushrooms over and cover.

7. Cook mushrooms until they're nice and tender

8. Remove mushrooms from the grill, and arrange on a platter.

Lobster and Shrimp Salad

1. Combine vinegar, mustard, honey, shallots and garlic in medium bowl.

2. Gradually whisk in oil.

3. Season dressing with salt and pepper.

4. In a large bowl, combine lobster, shrimp, mango, corn and microgreens.

5. Gradually pour dressing into lobster mixture until lightly coated.

6. Add more dressing, if desired.

7. Adjust seasonings.

8. Serve as a topping on the mushrooms.

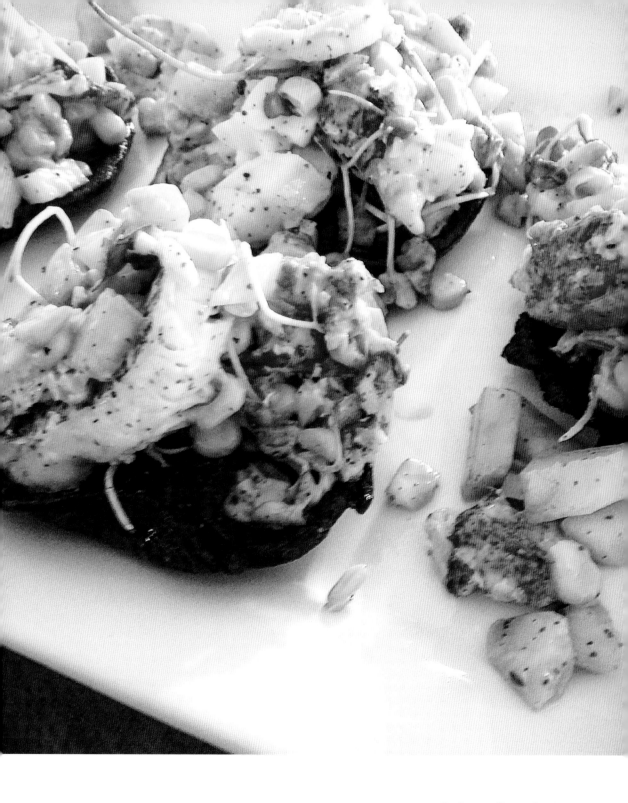

Roasted Sea Bass and Mushroom Broth with Quinoa, Sweet Potatoes and Kale

For Quinoa

3 tablespoons grape seed oil

½ small onion, diced

2 cloves garlic, minced

2 cups quinoa

4 cups chicken broth

Kosher salt fresh ground pepper

4 cups kale, stems removed and chopped

For Sweet Potatoes

2 tablespoons coconut oil

2 sweet potatoes, peeled and cut into
    ½-inch cubes

2 teaspoons maple syrup

 kosher salt and fresh ground black
    pepper

½ teaspoon grated nutmeg

½ teaspoon cumin

½ teaspoon cinnamon

For Sea Bass

1 tablespoon grape seed oil

Four 6-ounce skinless fillets of sea bass

Kosher salt freshly ground pepper

For Onions

1 yellow onion halved and sliced very
    thinly

½ teaspoon paprika

1 teaspoon Creole seasoning

1 ½ cups all-purpose flour

Canola oil for frying

For Mushroom Broth

1 pound button mushrooms

3 cloves garlic

3 sprigs fresh thyme

1 cup onions, chopped

4 cups cold water

2 pounds cremini mushrooms, washed,
    trimmed, and quartered

¼ cup grape seed oil

Kosher salt and freshly ground black pepper

Sweet potatoes

1. Preheat your oven to 350 degrees.

2. In a small saucepan, melt the coconut oil with the syrup over low heat.

3. Combine sweet potatoes, coconut oil mixture, salt, pepper and spices.

4. Spread the potatoes in an even layer on a large baking tray.

5. Roast, tossing occasionally to prevent burning until fork tender and caramelized.

6. Remove from the oven, and reserve until ready for use.

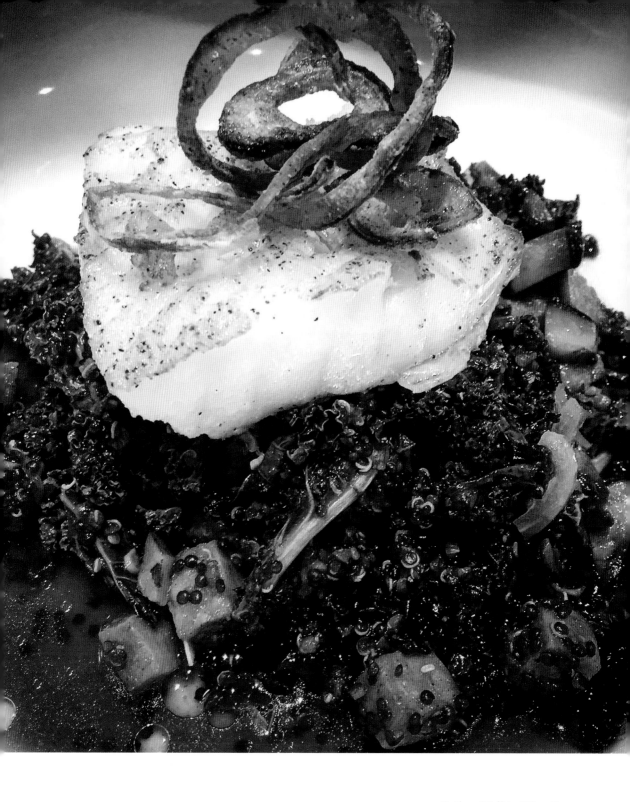

Quinoa

1. Heat one tablespoon of oil in a medium pot over medium-high heat, and sauté onions and garlic stirring often until softened.

2. Add the quinoa to the onion mixture, and stir to fully incorporate.

3. Add the broth, and season with salt and pepper.

4. Bring the mixture to a rolling boil, stirring occasionally.

5. Reduce the heat to low, cover and simmer until the quinoa has fully absorbed the liquid.

6. Remove quinoa from the heat, and set aside.

7. Heat the remaining two tablespoons of oil in a large sauté pan over medium-high heat.

8. Add the kale to the pan, and cook until it begins to wilt and reduce.

9. Season with salt and pepper.

10. In a large serving bowl, toss the cooked quinoa with the kale and sweet potatoes.

11. Adjust seasonings.

12. Spoon quinoa mixture in the center of a bowl.

Onions

1. Heat oil in a deep fat fryer.

2. Mix flour, paprika, and Creole seasoning in a medium bowl.

3. Thinly slice onion into rings.

4. Toss rings well in the flour mixture, shake off excess flour and deep fry until golden brown.

5. Drain well, and serve as a side dish or a tasty salad garnish.

Mushroom Broth

1. Preheat your oven to 375 degrees.

2. In a large saucepan, over medium-low heat simmer button mushrooms, garlic, thyme and onions in water for about an hour.

3. In a medium bowl, toss cremini mushrooms with grape seed oil, and season with salt and pepper.

4. Pour mushrooms on a foil-lined baking sheet, and spread into an even layer.

5. Roast mushrooms until they become soft.

6. Remove the mushrooms from the oven, and reserve until ready for use.

7. Strain broth into a separate pot through a fine strainer, and discard the solids.

8. Add roasted mushrooms to the broth, and simmer over medium heat for about 10 minutes. Adjust seasoning.

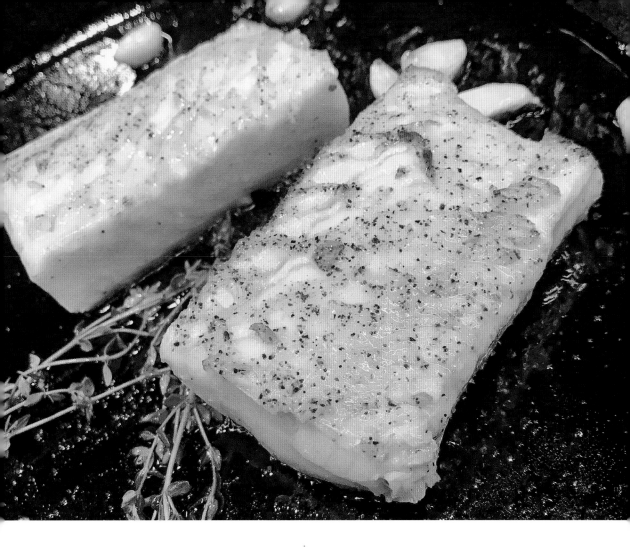

Sea Bass

1. Preheat your oven to 450 degrees.

2. Season fish with salt and pepper on both sides.

3. Heat oil in a large ovenproof pan over high heat.

4. Add fish and cook without moving, until fish is golden brown. This should take about three minutes.

5. Turn fish, transfer to oven and roast until they're just opaque in the center. This should take about five minutes.

6. Serve fish on the quinoa, ladle some broth on top and garnish with onions.

Collard Green and Blood Orange Salad with Candied Pecans and Creamy, Blood Orange Mustard Dressing

For Salad

2 bunches fresh collard greens

4 blood oranges peeled, and cut into ½ inch rounds

1 cup candied pecans

For Blood Orange Dressing

3 blood oranges, juiced

2 tablespoons red wine vinegar

2 tablespoons maple syrup

1 clove garlic, crushed

2 teaspoons Dijon mustard

Kosher salt and fresh ground pepper

¾ cup grape seed oil

Dressing

1. In a blender, combine the blood orange juice, red wine vinegar, maple syrup, garlic and Dijon mustard.

2. Blend until smooth.

3. With the blender running, add the grape seed oil in a steady stream until combined.

4. Taste, and season with salt and pepper.

Salad

1. Trim leaves from the tough stalks of collards.

2. Stack leaves, and roll up, starting at the long end.

3. Cut into thin slices.

4. Toss collards with ¼ cup of the dressing in a large bowl.

5. Cover and chill for 30 minutes.

6. Toss together blood orange slices and pecans with collard mixture.

7. Serve immediately.

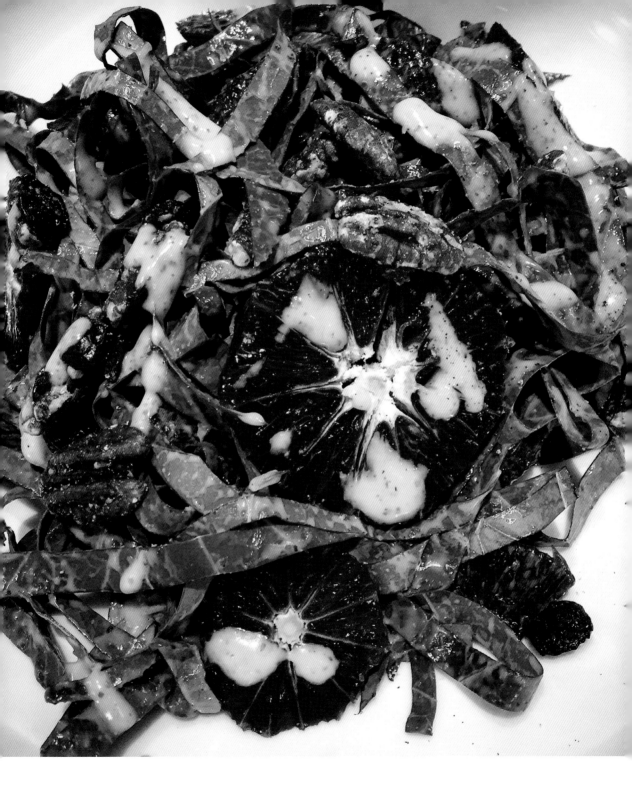

Grilled Peach and Bacon Salad with Buttermilk Vinaigrette

For Salad

3 peaches, pitted and each cut into
    6 wedges
Cooking spray
2 yellow onions, sliced into
    ½-inch rounds
10 cups trimmed arugula
6 pieces apple wood smoked bacon,
    cooked and cut into 1-inch pieces

For buttermilk dressing

½ cup buttermilk
1 cup yogurt
¼ cup sour cream
3 tablespoons rice wine vinegar
2 tablespoons apple juice
2 cloves garlic, minced
Kosher salt and freshly ground pepper

Buttermilk Vinaigrette

1. Whisk together all the ingredients in a medium bowl.

2. Season to taste with salt and pepper.

Salad

1. Prepare grill to high heat.

2. Place peach wedges on grill rack coated with cooking spray.

3. Grill 30 seconds on each side.

4. Remove peaches from grill, and set aside until ready for use.

5. Grill onions, season with salt and pepper while turning frequently until tender.

6. In a large bowl, combine greens, peaches, onions, bacon and dressing.

7. Toss until well coated.

8. Adjust seasonings, and serve.

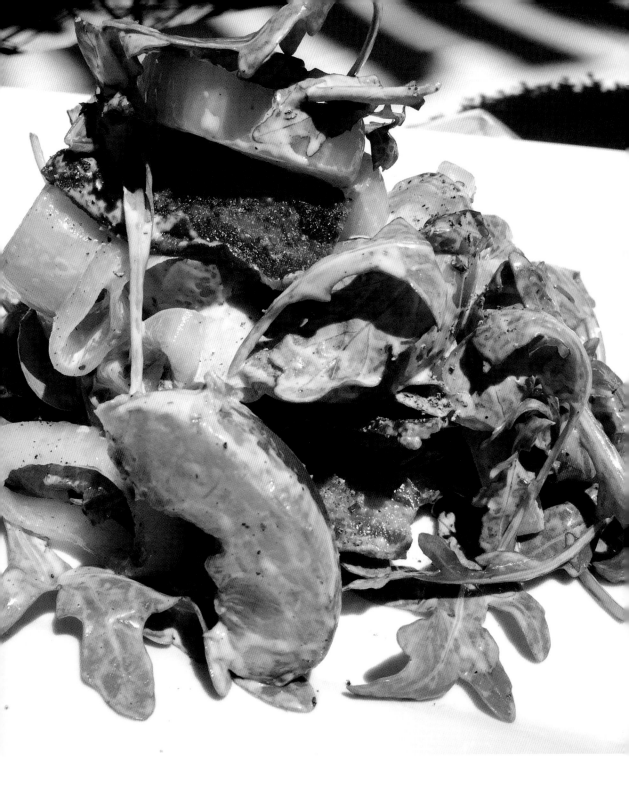

Shrimp and Noodle Bowl in Red Curry Broth

4 tablespoons coconut oil

½ pound medium shrimp, peeled and deveined

¼ cup yellow onion, thinly sliced

½ red bell pepper, sliced

½ orange bell pepper, sliced

¼ cup shiitake mushrooms, sliced

2 garlic cloves, minced

1 teaspoon freshly grated ginger

2 tablespoons red curry paste

¼ cup broccoli tops

2 cups unsweetened coconut milk

1 cup low-sodium chicken broth

1 tablespoon fish sauce

2 tablespoons fresh lime juice

1 cup rice noodles cooked

3 tablespoons fresh, chopped cilantro

2 green onions, sliced

Kosher salt and fresh ground pepper

1. Heat two tablespoons of the coconut oil over medium heat in a large sauté pan.

2. Add the shrimp to the pan, season with salt and pepper and cook until opaque.

3. Remove the shrimp from the pan, and reserve until ready for use.

4. Heat the remaining two tablespoons of coconut oil in a medium pot over medium heat.

5. Stir in the onions, peppers and mushrooms. Season with salt and pepper, and cook until the vegetables have slightly softened.

6. Add garlic, ginger and curry paste, and stir to fully incorporate.

7. Add coconut milk, broth, fish sauce and lime juice.

8. Bring the mixture to a boil then reduce the heat to low.

9. Add broccoli, shrimp, and cilantro, and simmer until broccoli is cooked and shrimp are warmed through. The broccoli should be bright green.

10. Place noodles in a bowl, and cover with the shrimp, vegetables and green onions.

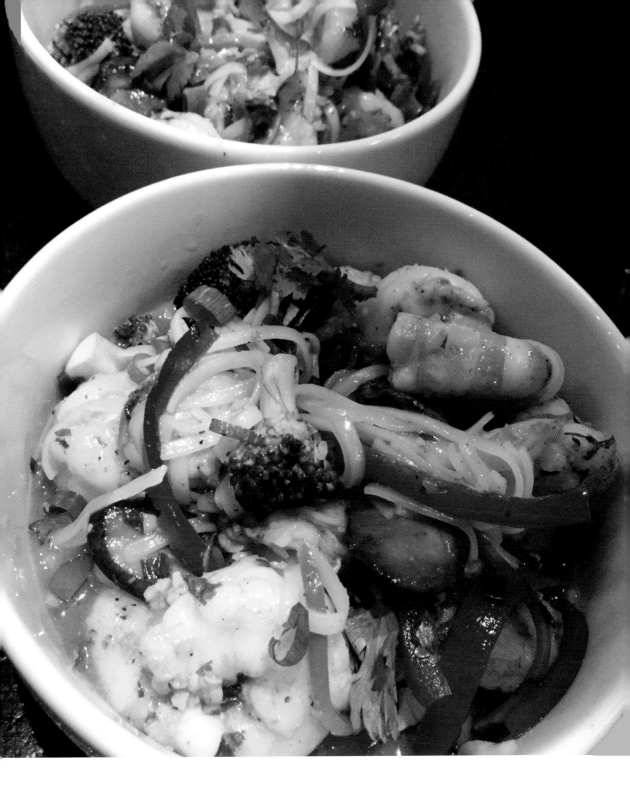

Prawns with Mandarin Slaw and Carrot Red Curry Dressing

For Prawns

6 giant prawns, with heads and shells on, butterflied and deveined

5 tablespoons grape seed oil

2 teaspoons five spice

4 garlic cloves, minced

1 teaspoon ginger, minced

1 teaspoon red pepper flakes

1 tablespoon ponzu

1/2 lime, sliced thin

Kosher salt and freshly ground pepper

For Slaw

4 tablespoons sesame oil

3 tablespoons fresh carrot juice

2 tablespoons fresh squeezed orange juice

1 tablespoon honey

1 tablespoon red curry paste

2 teaspoons ponzu

1 teaspoon grated ginger

1 garlic clove, minced

Kosher salt and fresh ground pepper

1 1/2 cups snow peas, cut on the diagonal into matchsticks

1 cup mandarin oranges

1/2 cup carrots cut into match sticks

1 red bell pepper, thinly sliced

1/2 cup cooked and shelled edamame

2 green onions, finely sliced

1/2 cup loosely packed, chopped fresh cilantro

Prawns

1. In a large bowl, combine prawns, three tablespoons grape seed oil, five spice, garlic, ginger, red pepper flakes, ponzu and lime.

2. Season with salt and pepper, and toss to coat evenly.

3. Marinate prawns for 30 minutes in the refrigerator.

4. Heat remaining grape seed oil in a large sauté pan over medium-high heat.

5. Remove the prawns from the marinade, and toss them into the pan.

6. Sauté for three minutes on each side until the shells are red and charred and prawns are cooked through.

Slaw

1. In a small bowl, whisk together sesame oil, orange juice, carrot juice, honey, red curry paste, ponzu, ginger and garlic.

2. Season with salt and pepper, and reserve until ready for use.

3. Combine all the slaw ingredients together in a medium-sized bowl.

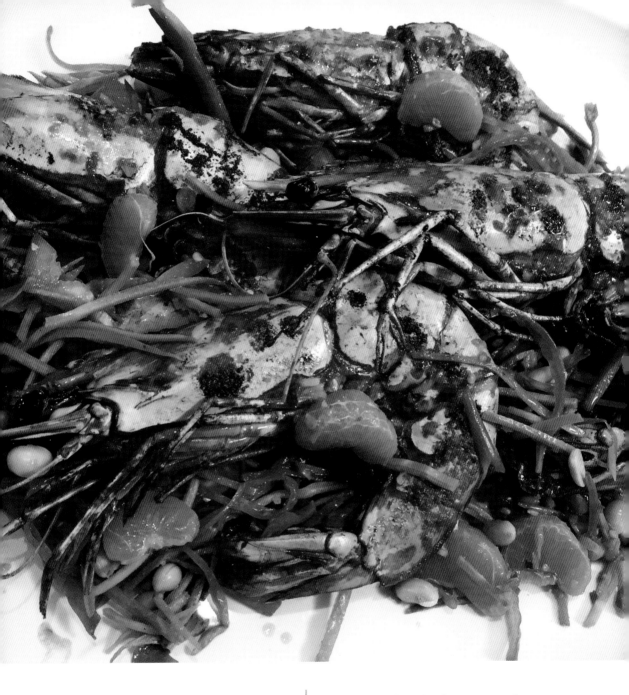

4. Pour the reserved dressing over the slaw, and toss to fully incorporate all the flavors.

5. Adjust seasonings.

6. Place slaw in the center of a platter, and top with sautéed prawns.

Mixed Field Greens with Granny Smith Apples, Mangos, Avocado, Toasted Almonds and Sesame Ginger Vinaigrette

For Salad

- 1 large mango, peeled, cut into 1-inch pieces
- 2 scallions, chopped
- 3 cups mixed greens
- 1 avocado, cut into 1-inch pieces
- ½ cup chopped cilantro
- ¼ cup mint leaves torn
- ¼ cup toasted almonds chopped, plus more for serving

For Sesame Ginger Dressing

- ¼ cup rice wine vinegar
- 1 teaspoon chopped fresh ginger
- 1½ tablespoons soy sauce
- 1 tablespoon honey
- 3 tablespoons toasted sesame oil
- 3 tablespoons grape seed oil
- Kosher salt and freshly ground pepper

For Sesame Ginger Dressing

1. Combine vinegar, ginger, soy sauce, honey, sesame oil and grape seed oil in a small bowl.

2. Whisk until fully incorporated.

3. Taste dressing, and adjust seasonings.

Salad

1. Combine mango, scallions, greens, avocado, cilantro, mint and almonds in a large bowl and toss.

2. Drizzle the dressing over the salad, and toss to coat.

3. Mound the salad in the center of a plate, and garnish with reserved almonds.

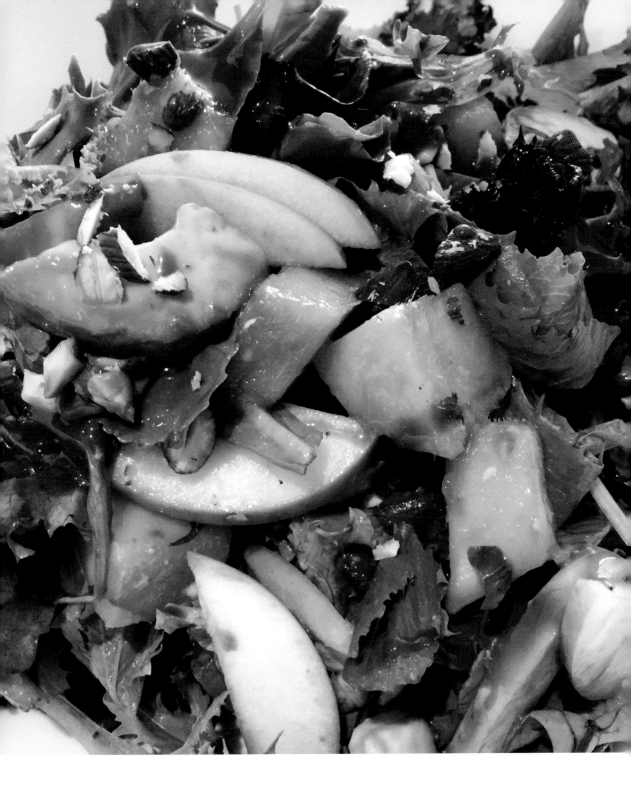

Heirloom Tomato and Watermelon Salad

For Salad

3 pounds medium and large mixed
   heirloom tomatoes, cut into ½
    -inch wedges

3 cups watermelon, seeded and cubed

2 kiwis, peeled, halved and sliced

1 ripe Hass avocado, chopped

¼ medium red onion, thinly sliced

¼ cup fresh lemon juice

1 garlic clove, minced

2 teaspoons agave

½ teaspoon ground coriander

¼ cup grape seed oil

3 tablespoons chopped, fresh cilantro

Kosher salt

1. In a large bowl, combine tomatoes, watermelon, kiwi, avocado and onion.

2. In a separate bowl, whisk together lemon juice, garlic, agave, coriander and grape seed oil.

3. Season with salt.

4. Pour vinaigrette over tomato mixture.

5. Fold in cilantro, and adjust seasonings.

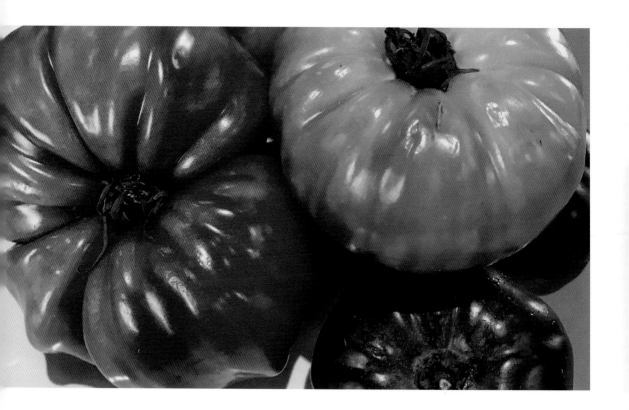

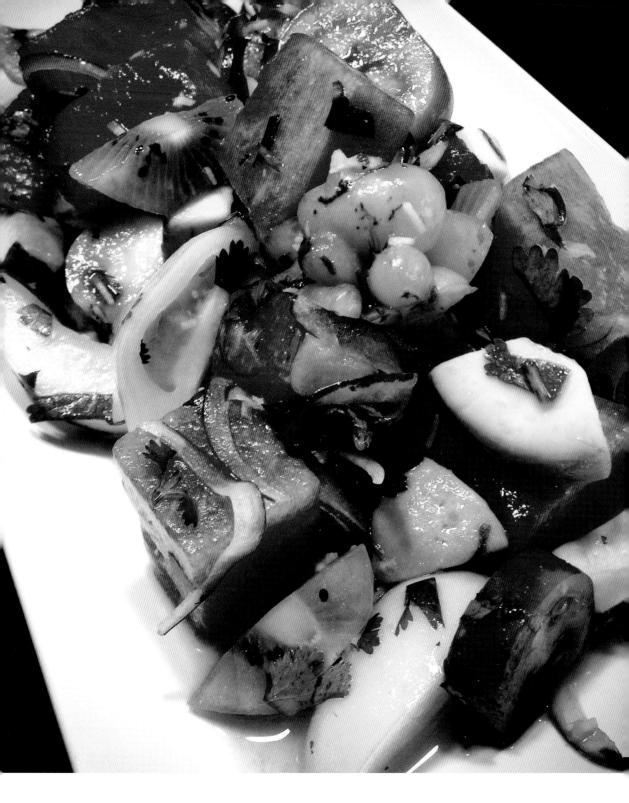

Grilled Jerk Lobster with Rum Raisin Mandarin Salsa

For Jerk Lobster

1 medium onion, chopped

3 medium scallions, chopped

1 Scotch bonnet pepper, chopped

3 garlic cloves, chopped

1 tablespoon five spice

1 tablespoon allspice berries, coarsely ground

1 tablespoon coarsely ground pepper

1 teaspoon dried thyme

1 teaspoon freshly grated nutmeg

1 teaspoon kosher salt

2 tablespoons orange juice

½ cup soy sauce

1 tablespoon canola oil

4 medium lobster tails, cleaned shell removed except the tail fin

For Salsa

½ cup golden raisins

3 tablespoons spiced rum

½ medium red onion, chopped

1 red bell pepper, seeded and chopped

1 teaspoon fresh ginger, minced

2 medium scallions, chopped

¼ cup cilantro

1 lime, juiced

1 tablespoon honey

1 cup fresh pineapple cut into ½-inch cubes

2 cups mandarin oranges, drained

Kosher salt and fresh ground pepper

Lobster

1. Light your grill.

2. Combine onion, scallions, scotch bonnet, garlic, five-spice powder, allspice, pepper, thyme, nutmeg and salt in a blender.

3. Blend until mixture is thick and fully incorporated.

4. With the blender running, add the orange juice, soy sauce and oil.

5. Brush the marinade over the lobster tails making sure they are fully coated.

6. Cover and refrigerate for 15-30 minutes.

7. Remove lobster tails from the refrigerator.

8. Grill the lobster over a medium-hot fire, turning occasionally, until well browned and cooked through. This should take about four to five minutes on each side. To prevent lobster tails from curling, insert water-soaked, wooden skewers into the tail lengthwise. Soaking the skewers in water also prevents them from burning while on the grill.

9. Transfer the jerk lobster to a platter.

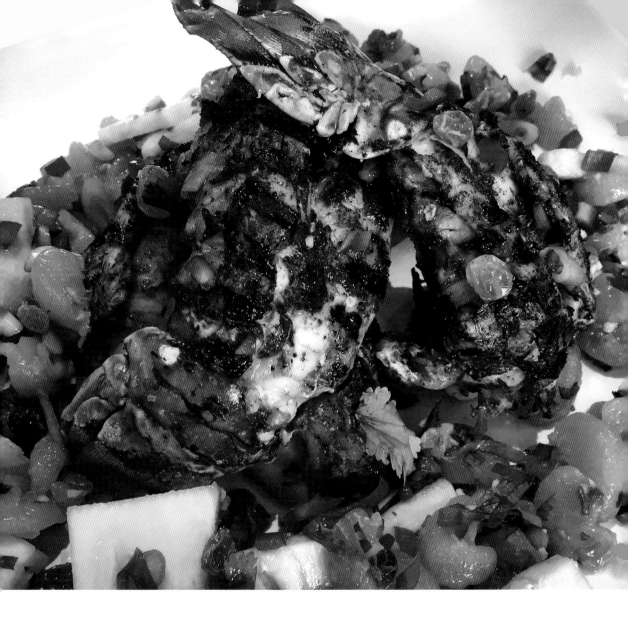

Salsa

1. In small bowl, combine raisins and rum.

2. Let raisins soak until they start to plump. This should take about an hour.

3. Drain, and reserve.

4. In a medium bowl, combine raisins, onion, bell pepper, ginger, scallions, cilantro, lime juice, honey, pineapple and mandarins.

5. Toss, and season with salt and pepper.

6. Use to dress the lobster.

Shrimp with Spinach and Balsamic-Roasted Mushrooms

For Spinach

3 tablespoons grape seed oil

1 tablespoon unsalted butter

1 pound large shrimp, peeled and deveined

1 ½ teaspoons Creole seasoning

½ small red onion, sliced thin

2 garlic cloves, finely chopped

½ yellow bell pepper, seeded and sliced

3 bunches spinach, cleaned and stems trimmed

3 portobello mushrooms, roasted and sliced

Kosher salt and freshly ground black pepper

For Mushrooms

4 portobello mushrooms, stemmed and gills removed

¼ cup extra-virgin olive oil

¼ cup fig balsamic vinegar (regular balsamic is fine, too)

1 tablespoon fresh thyme

1 ½ teaspoons red pepper flakes

Kosher salt and fresh ground pepper

Mushrooms

1. Preheat your oven to 400 degrees.

2. Combine olive oil, balsamic vinegar and fresh thyme in a small bowl.

3. Brush both sides of the mushrooms liberally with the balsamic mixture. You want to get it all over the mushrooms.

4. Put the mushrooms on a rimmed baking sheet stem side up, and season with salt and pepper.

5. Bake until the mushrooms have shrunk down and softened. This usually takes 10 to 12 minutes.

6. Remove the baking sheet from the oven, and slice the mushrooms. Don't discard the cooking juices they're full of flavor. We'll use them later.

Spinach

1. In a large sauté pan over medium high heat, melt butter with one tablespoon of grape seed oil. Combining the two will prevent the butter from burning too quickly.

2. Add the shrimp to the pan.

3. Add the Creole seasoning, and stir frequently until shrimp are bright pink and opaque.

4. Remove the shrimp from the pan, and reserve until ready for use.

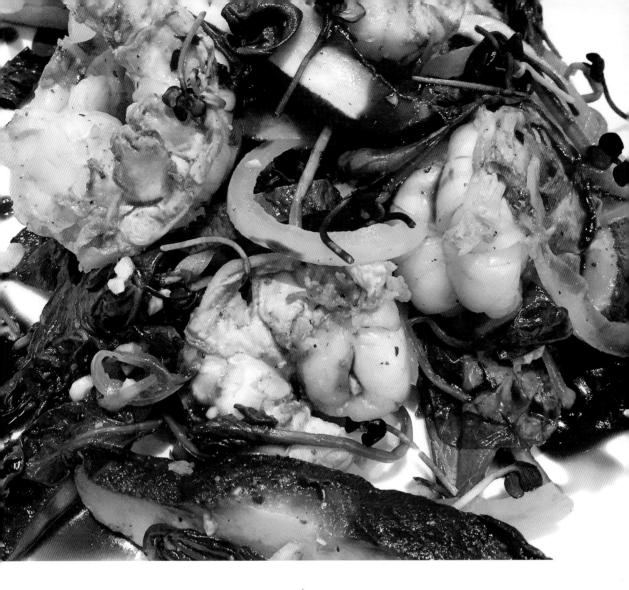

5. Add remaining two tablespoons grape seed oil to the pan over medium-high heat.

6. Add onions, garlic and bell pepper stirring until fragrant and vegetables soften.

7. Add spinach, season with salt and pepper and toss until the leaves begin to wilt.

8. Add in mushrooms, reserved shrimp and reserved mushroom juices, and toss until tender. This should take about two minutes.

9. Adjust seasoning, and serve immediately.

Coffee-Rubbed Bison Ribeye and Moros y Cristianos Tacos

For Steaks

2 boneless bison ribeye steaks

¼ cup ground espresso

2 tablespoons smoked paprika

2 tablespoons freshly ground
   black pepper

2 tablespoons dark brown sugar

1 tablespoon chili powder

1 teaspoon cumin

1 teaspoon ground ginger

1 ½ teaspoons mustard powder

2 tablespoons grape seed oil

Canola or olive oil

Kosher salt and coarsely ground
   black pepper

For Moros y Cristianos

2 tablespoons grape seed oil

4 cloves garlic, minced

1 medium yellow onion, chopped

1 green pepper, seeded and chopped

1 bay leaf

1 teaspoon smoked paprika

¼ teaspoon ground cumin

½ teaspoon dried oregano

1 cup long-grain brown rice

2 cans black beans, not drained

2 cups low-sodium chicken broth

Kosher salt and fresh ground pepper

For Chipotle Aioli

1 cup avocado mayonnaise

1 teaspoon fresh lime juice

1 garlic clove, minced

½ teaspoon agave

2 tablespoons Chipotle in adobo

Kosher salt and fresh ground pepper

Moros y Cristianos

1. In a medium pot over medium-high heat, sauté the onion, garlic and green pepper in two tablespoons grape seed oil stirring until vegetables are softened and translucent.

2. Season with salt and pepper.

3. Add the bay leaf, smoked paprika, cumin, oregano and rice. Stir until well mixed and all the rice is coated in oil.

4. Add the beans, their liquid and chicken broth to the pot. Cover and bring to a boil then reduce to a simmer for 35 to 40 minutes, or until all the liquid has been absorbed by the rice.

5. Allow the covered pot to sit off the heat to steam.

6. Fluff the rice with a fork, and hold until ready for use.

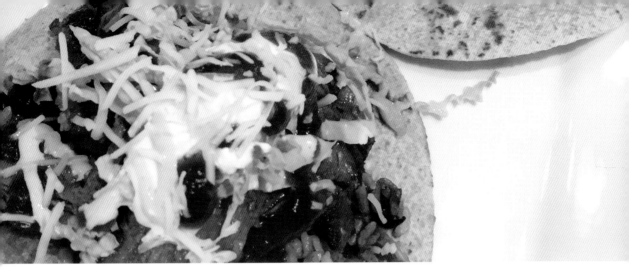

Steaks

1. Preheat your oven to 400 degrees.

2. Combine espresso, paprika, pepper, brown sugar, chili powder, cumin, ginger and mustard in a small bowl.

3. Set a wire rack inside a large rimmed baking sheet.

4. Season steaks with kosher salt and spice rub. Be sure to press the rub into all sides of the entire surface of the steak.

5. Heat two tablespoons grape seed oil in a large cast-iron skillet over high heat.

6. Place steak in skillet. Sear steak for one minute. Any longer and the rub will start to burn.

7. Turn steak over, and sear for one minute.

8. Transfer steaks to a baking sheet and cook in the oven to medium-rare doneness. This normally takes about eight to 10 minutes.

9. Remove the pan from the oven, and let the steaks rest five minutes before slicing.

Aioli

1. Put mayonnaise, lime juice, garlic, agave and chipotle in a food processor or blender.

2. Blend until fully incorporated and smooth.

3. Taste, and season with salt and pepper.

4. Store in an air-tight container in refrigerator until ready to use.

Assembly

1. Spoon Moros y Cristianos in the center of the tortilla.

2. Top with sliced ribeye followed by shredded lettuce, cheese, taco sauce and aioli.

Roasted Salmon with Sriracha Honey Glaze and Baby Kale Salad

For Salmon

Four 6-ounce salmon fillets

2 teaspoons five spice

Kosher salt and fresh ground pepper

1/3 cup honey

1/3 cup Sriracha sauce

1 tablespoon seasoned rice vinegar

2 teaspoons ponzu

1/4 teaspoon sesame oil

For Baby Kale Salad

6 cups baby kale

1/4 cup cilantro, chopped

1 cup fresh blueberries

2 oranges, supremed
    (instructions on p.64)

1/4 cup toasted sesame oil

2 tablespoons soy sauce

2 tablespoons orange juice

1 tablespoon honey

1 teaspoon fish sauce

2 teaspoons Sriracha

Kosher salt and black pepper

Salad

1. In a large bowl, combine kale, cilantro, blueberries and orange segments.

2. In a medium bowl, whisk together sesame oil, soy sauce, orange juice, honey, fish sauce and Sriracha.

3. Season with salt and pepper.

4. Drizzle dressing over salad while gently tossing.

Salmon

1. Preheat your oven to 350 degrees.

2. Season salmon with five spice and salt and pepper.

3. In a small bowl, whisk together the honey, Sriracha, rice vinegar and ponzu.

4. Heat the grape seed oil in a large nonstick ovenproof pan over high heat.

5. Add seasoned salmon to the skillet skin side up.

6. Cook until golden.

7. Turn the salmon, and spoon the glaze on top.

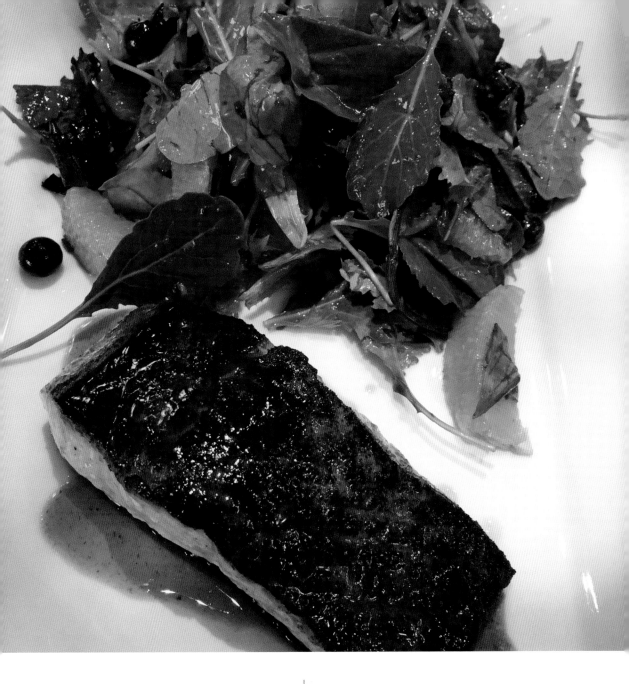

8. Transfer the pan to the oven, and bake the salmon until cooked through.

9. Remove salmon from the oven, and transfer to plates.

10. Drizzle salmon with remaining glaze, and serve with baby kale salad.

Crab and Shrimp Cake with Southern Style Succotash and Curry Ponzu Emulsion

For Crab and Shrimp Cake

2 eggs, beaten

½ cup avocado mayonnaise

¼ teaspoon cayenne pepper

1 teaspoon smoked paprika

½ teaspoon dry mustard

1 teaspoon Creole seasoning

1 tablespoon Worcestershire sauce

1 pound jumbo lump crabmeat, drained and picked

4 ounces cooked shrimp, chopped

½ cup yellow onion, finely chopped

¼ cup red bell pepper, finely chopped

1 tablespoon fresh thyme

½ cup gluten free panko bread crumbs

grape seed oil for frying

For Succotash

2 tablespoons grape seed oil

1 small red onion, chopped

2 garlic cloves, minced

1 teaspoon Creole seasoning

½ teaspoon smoked paprika

1 ½ cups fresh corn

1 teaspoon red pepper flakes

1 ½ cups frozen, baby lima beans

½ pound fresh okra, tops removed and sliced length wise

2 cups fire-roasted tomatoes, canned

2 tablespoons apple cider vinegar

2 teaspoons fresh thyme

Kosher salt and fresh ground pepper

For Curry Ponzu Emulsion

1 tablespoon unsalted butter

1 shallot, sliced

½ teaspoon fresh ginger, minced

½ pear peeled, cored and thinly sliced

2 cloves garlic, minced

1 bay leaf

2 sprigs fresh thyme

1 tablespoon curry powder

1 teaspoon turmeric

1 ½ teaspoon ponzu

1/4 cup chicken stock

½ cup coconut milk

Kosher salt and freshly ground pepper

Crab Cakes

1. Combine eggs, mayonnaise, pepper, paprika, mustard, Creole seasoning and Worcestershire sauce in a medium mixing bowl.

2. Mix thoroughly to fully incorporate flavors.

3. In a separate bowl, combine crabmeat, shrimp, onions, peppers, thyme and bread crumbs.

4. Add wet mix to crab mixture, and fold in.

5. Portion crab mix into patties, and refrigerate 15 minutes to let set.

6. Heat oil in a medium cast-iron skillet over medium heat.

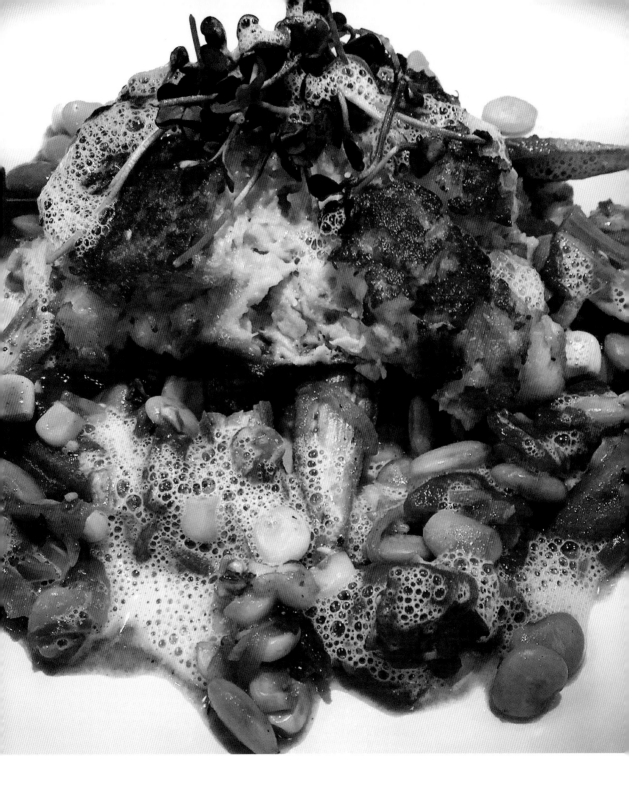

7. Cook patties until golden brown on both sides. This should take about two minutes on each side.

8. Drain on a paper towel lined pan.

Curry Emulsion

1. Melt the butter over medium heat in a medium saucepan.

2. Add shallots, garlic, ginger, pear, bay leaf and thyme.

3. Stir until the vegetables are soft.

4. Stir in curry powder, turmeric, ponzu and stock.

5. Reduce heat and simmer for about five minutes.

6. Add coconut milk, and bring to a boil for about one minute.

7. Reduce heat, and remove bay leaf and thyme.

8. Pour sauce into a blender, and blend until smooth.

9. Strain the mixture.

10. If sauce is too thick, it can be thinned out by adding more stock.

11. Season with salt and freshly ground pepper.

12. Keep warm until ready for use.

Succotash

1. Heat oil in a medium cast-iron skillet over high heat.

2. Add onions to skillet, and stir until softened.

3. Add garlic, Creole seasoning and paprika.

4. Stir continuously.

5. Add corn, red pepper flakes, lima beans, okra, and tomatoes until vegetables are tender.

6. Add vinegar and fresh thyme. Season with salt and pepper to taste.

7. Using a hand blender, foam curry sauce until it is frothy.

8. Spoon succotash in the center of a serving plate. Top with a crab and shrimp cake, and drizzle with curry emulsion.

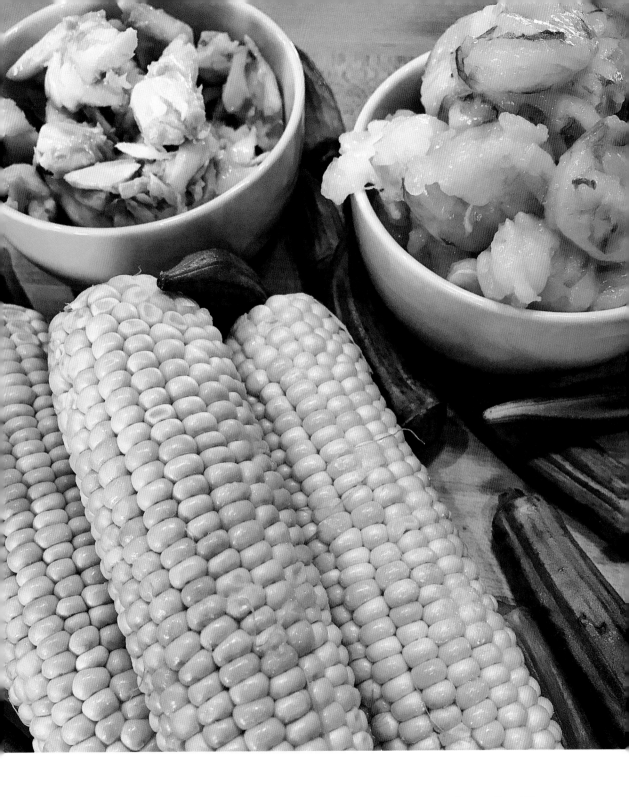

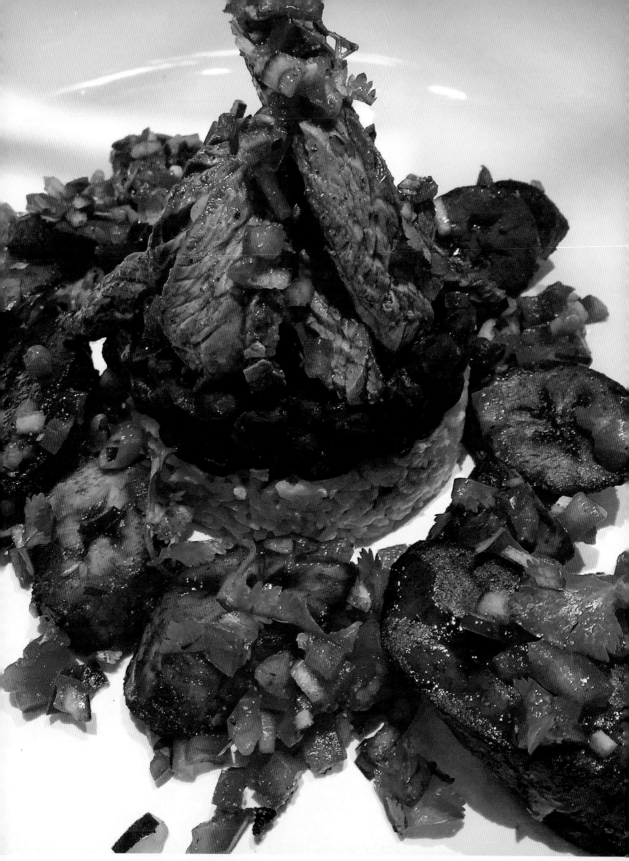

Dinner

My mother would come home from a hard day of teaching and start cooking right away. It was our time to discuss our day. It also provided me with another opportunity to inadvertently learn how to cook.

Dinner provides sustenance not only for the body but for the mind as well through good food and conversation.

Eating Dinner to Win

Try eating a vegetable-packed salad before your main course. Doing this will help you cut your overall calorie intake during dinner.

Miso Roasted Sea Bass with Ginger Garlic Broccoli Rabe

For Sea Bass

Four 6-ounce sea bass fillets

1/3 cup sake

1/3 cup mirin

2 teaspoons ginger juice

1/3 cup light miso

3 tablespoons brown sugar

2 tablespoons ponzu

For Broccoli Rabe

3 bunches broccoli rabe

3 tablespoons grape seed oil

4 garlic cloves, sliced

3 teaspoons fresh ginger, minced

1/2 teaspoon crushed red pepper flakes

Kosher salt and freshly ground pepper

Sea Bass

1. Mix sake, mirin, ginger, miso, brown sugar and ponzu in a small bowl.

2. Place sea bass in a large Ziploc bag.

3. Pour all but two tablespoons of the miso marinade over the sea bass, and refrigerate overnight.

4. Remove the sea bass from the marinade, and wipe off any excess marinade.

5. Preheat oven to 400 degrees.

6. Preheat an outdoor grill or stovetop grill plate.

7. Place the fish on the grill, and lightly grill on both sides until the surface caramelizes.

8. Transfer the fish fillets to a rimmed baking sheet.

9. Place the sea bass in the oven, and bake until just opaque in center. This typically takes about eight to 10 minutes.

Broccoli Rabe

1. Cut off and discard the tough ends of the broccoli rabe, and cut the rest of into two-inch pieces.

2. Bring a large pot of water to a boil.

3. Cook broccoli rabe in boiling water until al dente.

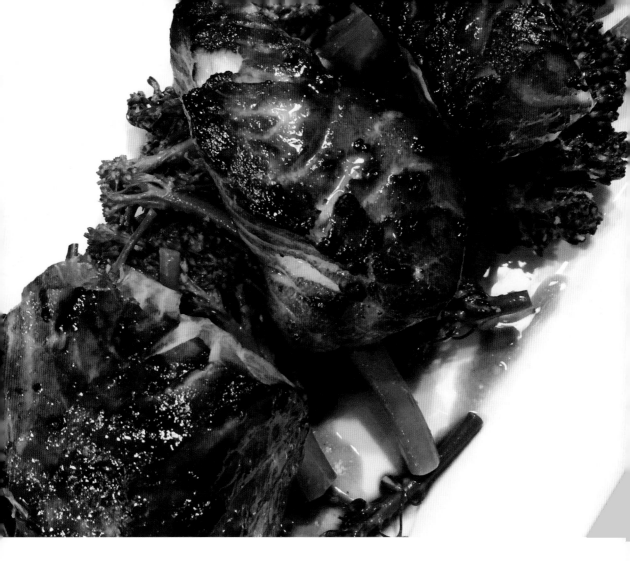

4. Drain and shock the broccoli rabe by plunging it into ice water bath. This will stop the broccoli rabe from continuing to cook.

5. Drain the broccoli rabe well.

6. Heat the grape seed oil in a large skillet over medium-high heat.

7. Add broccoli rabe, ginger, red pepper flakes and garlic, and stir until thoroughly heated.

8. Remove from heat, and season with salt and pepper.

9. Arrange broccoli rabe on a serving platter, and top with sea bass.

10. Finish by drizzling reserved marinade over the sea bass.

Eggplant Cannoli

For Eggplant

2 medium eggplants, cut lengthwise
into ½-inch slices

Grape seed oil cooking spray

For Sauce

2 tablespoons grape seed oil

3 large shallots, sliced

4 cloves garlic, minced

2 cans fire-roasted diced tomatoes

Juice of 1 orange (about ½ cup)

½ tablespoon dried thyme

2 teaspoons curry powder

Kosher salt and fresh ground pepper

For Cannoli Filling

½ pound Italian turkey sausage,
removed from the casing and cooked

2 cloves garlic, minced

2 cups kale, stems removed

¼ cup smoked, sun-dried tomatoes

8 ounces smoked Gouda

8 ounces ricotta

Sauce

1. Heat oil in a medium skillet over medium heat.

2. Cook shallots and garlic until soft.

3. Reduce heat, and continue cooking until golden.

4. Next add tomatoes, orange juice, thyme, salt, pepper and curry.

5. Bring sauce to a boil then lower heat and simmer uncovered until sauce has thickened.

6. Adjust seasonings. Remove from the heat, and let cool.

Eggplant

1. Heat your oven to 400 degrees.

2. Liberally spray a baking sheet with oil.

3. Place slices of the eggplant on the baking sheet without overlapping.

4. Generously oil the slices, flip and oil the other side.

5. Season with salt and pepper.

6. Bake for about 10 minutes, and then flip each of the slices over. Continue baking until the slices start to turn a golden brown.

7. While the eggplant slices bake, sauté the chopped kale with the garlic in a medium sauté pan over medium-high heat until wilted.

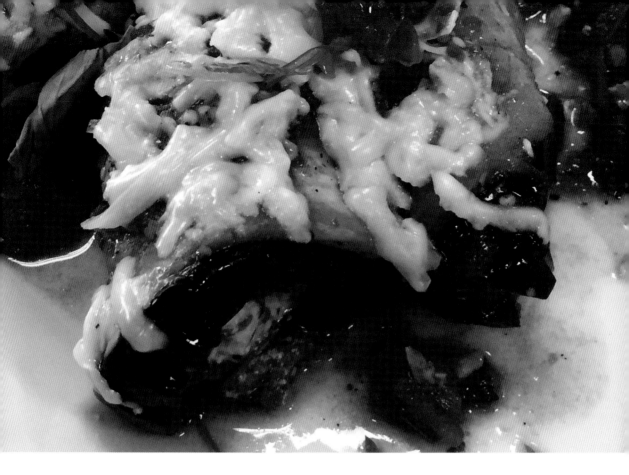

8. Remove eggplant from the oven, and let cool for about five minutes.

9. Reduce oven heat to 350 degrees.

10. Next combine the ricotta, four ounces of Gouda, kale, sun-dried tomatoes and sausage in a large bowl, and mix until everything is evenly distributed.

11. Adjust seasonings.

12. Spoon half of the sauce into the bottom of a baking dish.

13. Place about two tablespoons of the filling onto the cut end of an eggplant, and roll it up.

14. Place the cannoli in the baking dish, and repeat until all of the eggplant has been used.

15. Top the rolls with more of the sauce and the remaining Gouda.

16. Place the cannoli in the oven. Cook until heated through, and cheese is melted.

Lobster and Shrimp Cobb Salad with Dijon Vinaigrette

For Salad

- 1 tablespoon grape seed oil
- 1 tablespoon unsalted butter
- 3 teaspoons Creole seasoning
- 1 teaspoon curry powder
- 1 teaspoon smoked paprika
- 4 medium lobster tails, shells removed except for the tail fin
- 1 pound jumbo shrimp, peeled and deveined except for the tail fin
- 6 cups mixed field greens
- 6 hard-boiled eggs, peeled and quartered
- 2 avocados, halved, pitted and cubed
- 1 ½ cups heirloom cherry tomatoes, halved
- 1 ½ cups green beans, cook and cooled
- ¼ cup capers, drained
- Salt and freshly cracked black pepper
- 1 cup asiago cheese, shaved

For Dijon Vinaigrette

- ½ cup rice wine vinegar
- 2 tablespoons Dijon mustard
- 3 tablespoons honey
- 2 garlic cloves
- 1 cup canola
- ¼ cup extra-virgin olive oil
- Kosher salt fresh ground pepper

Lobster and Shrimp

1. Heat the butter with the grape seed oil in a large sauté pan over medium-high heat.

2. Once butter is melted and starts to bubble, reduce heat to medium.

3. Add in the lobster tails and shrimp.

4. Season with Creole seasoning, curry powder and paprika, and continue to cook while stirring until done. Normally, this takes about four to five minutes.

5. Remove from the pan, and let cool until ready for use.

Dijon Vinaigrette

1. Combine rice wine vinegar, Dijon mustard, honey and garlic in a blender.

2. Blend until all ingredients are well incorporated.

3. Slowly add canola and olive oil in a steady stream while the motor is still running.

4. Season with salt and pepper, and reserve until ready for use.

Salad

1. In a large bowl, combine salad greens, eggs, avocados, tomatoes, green beans, capers and ½ of the cheese.

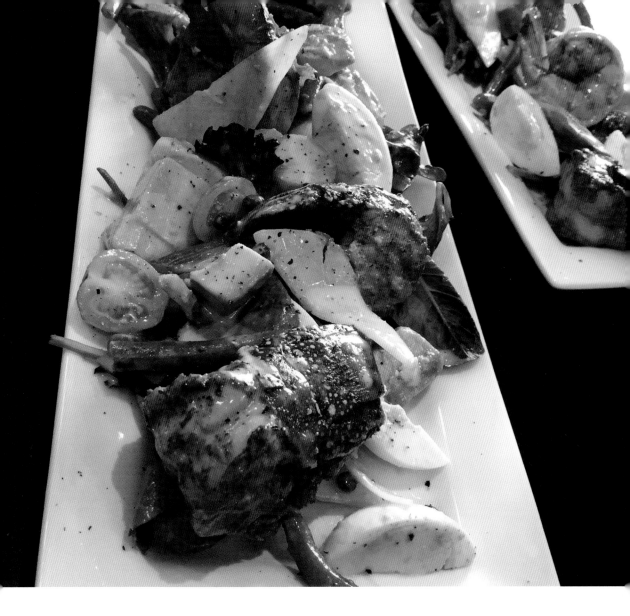

2. Gently toss the salad with some of the Dijon vinaigrette. Start with about ⅓ cup of the dressing. Feel free to add more.

3. Season with salt and pepper.

4. Arrange salad in the center of the plate.

5. Place lobster tail and shrimp around salad.

6. Drizzle a little dressing over the lobster and shrimp.

7. Garnish with shaved asiago.

Garlic Shrimp in a White Bean Ragu

1 pound large, peeled and deveined
  shrimp

4 tablespoons grape seed oil, divided

1 1/2 teaspoons smoked paprika

1/2 teaspoon cumin

4 garlic cloves, minced and divided

1 teaspoon red pepper flakes

1 bay leaf

3 sprigs fresh thyme

1 can fire-roasted, diced tomatoes,
  drained

1 tablespoon tomato paste

2 cans (about 15 ounces each) white
  beans, rinsed and drained

1 cup low-sodium chicken broth

1 teaspoon truffle honey

Kosher salt and fresh ground pepper

1. In a medium bowl, season shrimp with smoked paprika, cumin, salt and pepper.

2. Heat two tablespoons of the grape seed oil in a large skillet over medium-high heat.

3. Add shrimp to skillet, sauté until just cooked through. Place shrimp into a bowl and set aside until ready for use.

4. Return the skillet to heat, and add remaining oil.

5. Next heat garlic, pepper flakes, bay leaf and sauté until fragrant.

6. Add tomatoes and cook until most of the liquid evaporates.

7. Add in tomato paste, and cook until mixture starts to darken.

8. Add beans, broth and thyme.

9. Simmer until a thick consistency is reached.

10. Return shrimp to the pan, and cook until just heated through.

11. Adjust seasonings.

12. Drizzle with truffle honey and serve.

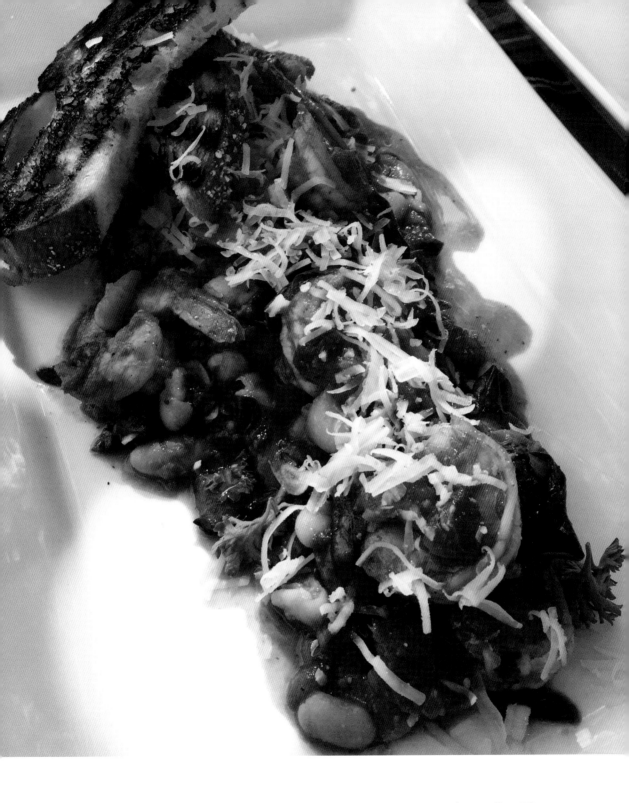

Chicken Quinoa and Roasted Sweet Potato Lasagna with Smoked Gouda and Cheddar

For Chicken Quinoa

3 cups sweet potatoes, diced

1 teaspoon Creole seasoning

1 teaspoon cumin

1 teaspoon cinnamon

2 tablespoons grape seed oil

1/4 cup red onion, minced

1 garlic clove, minced

1 teaspoon dried oregano

2 cups low-sodium chicken broth

1 cup quinoa

2 cups tomato sauce

8 cloves of garlic

2 medium chicken breasts, cooked and chopped

2 cups zucchini, sliced

1 1/2 cups smoked Gouda, shredded

1/2 cup white cheddar, shredded

For Tomato Sauce

2 tablespoons grape seed oil

3 large shallots, sliced

4 cloves garlic, minced

2 cans fire-roasted, diced tomatoes

Juice of 1 orange (about 1/2 cup)

1/2 tablespoon dried thyme

2 teaspoons curry powder

Kosher salt and fresh ground pepper

Sauce

1. Heat oil in a medium skillet over medium heat.

2. Cook shallots and garlic until soft.

3. Reduce heat, and continue cooking until golden brown.

4. Add tomatoes, orange juice, thyme, salt, pepper and curry.

5. Bring sauce to a boil then lower heat and simmer uncovered until sauce has thickened.

6. Adjust seasonings, remove from heat and let cool.

Lasagna

1. Preheat the oven to 350, and lightly grease a casserole dish with cooking spray.

2. Toss sweet potatoes with Creole seasoning, cumin, cinnamon and one tablespoon of grape seed oil. Then roast on a large baking sheet for 25 to 30 minutes.

3. Heat the remaining one tablespoon of grape seed oil in a medium saucepan over medium-high heat.

4. Add red onion, garlic, and oregano, and stir frequently until softened and fragrant.

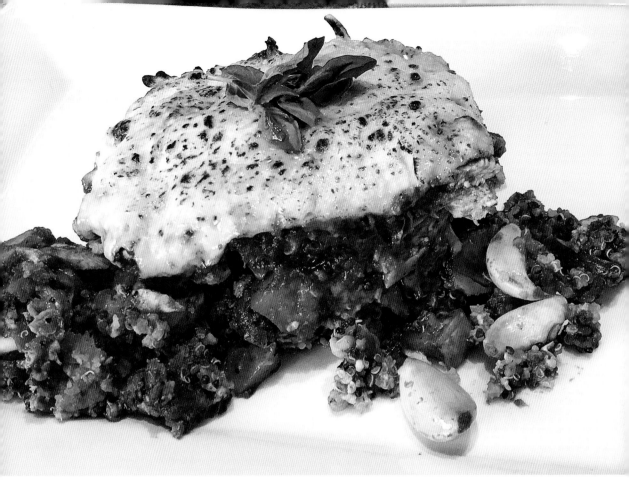

5. Add chicken broth, and bring to a boil.

6. Stir in quinoa, reduce to a simmer, cover and cook for 15 minutes. Fluff and set aside until ready for use.

7. Spread about 1/3 cup of the sauce on the bottom of the casserole dish.

8. Spread cooked quinoa over the sauce.

9. Add garlic cloves on top of quinoa then top with more sauce.

10. Make a layer of all the zucchini then the sweet potatoes, and add more sauce.

11. Add the chopped chicken, and end with the remainder of the tomato sauce.

12. Spread the smoked Gouda and white cheddar cheeses evenly on top.

13. Bake lasagna until it's heated through, and the cheese is bubbling and slightly browned on top.

Zucchini Pasta with Clams and Scallops

10 large scallops

2 ½ tablespoons unsalted butter

1 tablespoon extra-virgin olive oil

3 garlic cloves, sliced

1 shallot, minced

1 teaspoon red pepper flakes

1 cup cherry tomatoes, sliced

1/2 teaspoon Dijon mustard

¼ cup clam juice

½ cup dry white wine

Kosher salt freshly ground black pepper

2 pounds clams, rinsed and scrubbed

4 cups spiralized zucchini

1. Season scallops with salt and pepper.

2. Melt 1 ½ tablespoons unsalted butter in a large saucepan over medium-high heat.

3. Add scallops, and cook until golden brown on both sides.

4. Remove the saucepan from the heat, and transfer scallops to a plate. Set aside until ready for use. Don't clean saucepan.

5. Place the large saucepan back over medium heat, and add the olive oil.

6. Add the garlic and shallots, and cook until the shallots have softened.

7. Add the red pepper flakes, cherry tomatoes, Dijon mustard, clam juice and wine. Season to taste.

8. Bring sauce to a boil then reduce the heat to low.

9. Simmer sauce until it has reduced by half.

10. Add the clams to the sauce, and cover.

11. Steam clams until they open. Discard any clams that don't open.

12. Stir in the zucchini noodles and one tablespoon of butter.

13. Cook zucchini pasta for two to three minutes or until al dente.

14. Add in reserved scallops, and cook.

15. Divide the pasta among bowls, and serve.

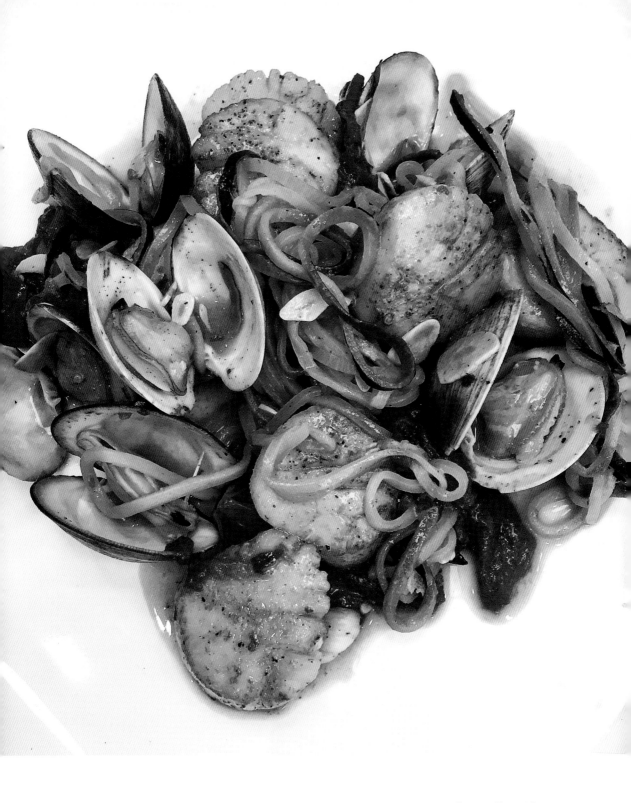

Grilled Bison Skirt Steak with Black Beans, Yellow Rice and Plaintain Salsa

For Skirt Steak

2 pounds bison skirt steak

Kosher salt and fresh ground pepper

For Black Beans

1 tablespoon grape seed oil

½ medium red onion, chopped

2 garlic cloves, finely chopped

1 large jalapeño, seeded and chopped

2 teaspoons ground cumin

1 teaspoon smoked paprika

3 bay leaves

2 cans black beans, rinsed and drained

1 ½ cups low-sodium chicken broth

1 teaspoon balsamic vinegar

Kosher salt and fresh ground pepper

For Yellow Rice

1 tablespoon unsalted butter

1 teaspoon ground turmeric

¼ teaspoon ground cumin

¼ teaspoon cinnamon

1 cup long grain brown rice

3 ¼ cups low-sodium chicken broth

Kosher salt and freshly ground pepper

For Plantain Salsa

2 very ripe plantains (It's okay if they're black as long the inside isn't moldy or super mushy.)

1 tablespoon of coconut oil

1 small red onion, diced

1 cup tomatoes, diced

2 green onions, chopped

¼ cup chopped fresh cilantro

1 jalapeñoo, minced

3 tablespoons fresh lime juice

1 tablespoon honey

Kosher salt

Black Beans

1. In a large saucepan, warm oil over medium-high heat.

2. Add onion, garlic, jalapeño, cumin, smoked paprika and bay leaves, and sauté until onions soften.

3. Add beans and chicken broth, and stir occasionally.

4. Continue cooking until thick, stirring frequently for about 10 minutes.

5. Stir in balsamic vinegar and season with salt and pepper. Transfer to bowl, and keep warm.

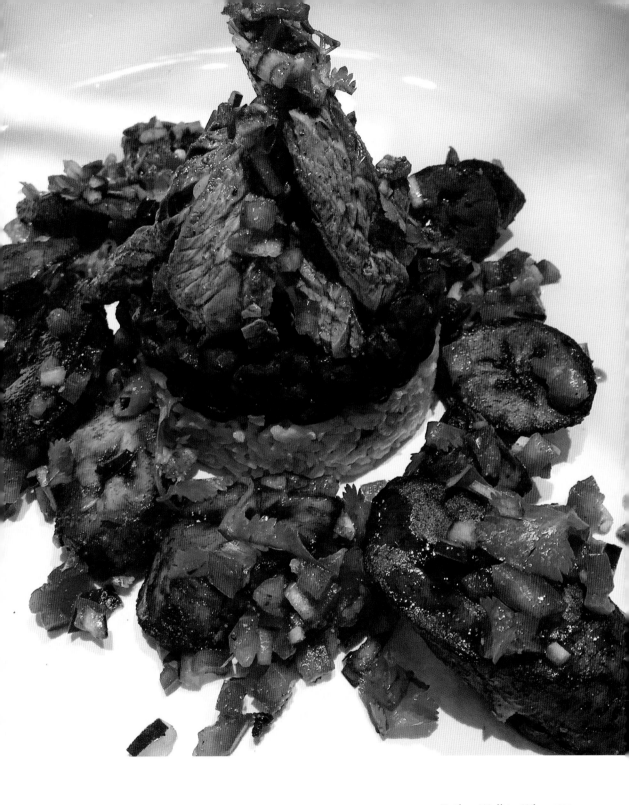

Yellow Rice

1. Melt butter in a medium saucepan over medium heat.

2. Stir in the turmeric, cumin and cinnamon, and heat until fragrant.

3. Add in the brown rice, and stir to make sure every grain is coated with the butter and spices.

4. Pour the broth over the rice, season with salt and pepper and bring to a boil.

5. Reduce heat to a simmer, and cover.

6. Cook rice until the broth is absorbed, and the rice is tender.

7. Remove from the heat and let sit, covered, without stirring.

8. Fluff with a fork, and reserve until ready for use.

Plantain Salsa

1. Preheat your oven to 400 degrees.

2. Cut ripe plantains on the diagonal into 1/2-inch thick slices.

3. Place the plantain slices in a medium bowl with the coconut oil and toss to coat.

4. Arrange the plantain slices on a baking sheet, and bake.

5. Turn plantains after the first 15 minutes.

6. Cook for an additional 10 minutes, or until well caramelized on both sides.

7. In a large bowl, combine red onion, tomatoes, green onions, cilantro, jalapeño, lime juice and honey.

8. Gently toss, and adjust seasonings.

9. Gently fold in plantains.

Skirt Steak

1. Season skirt steak with salt and ground pepper.

2. Heat grill to high.

3. Cook skirt steak until medium rare, or until an instant-read thermometer shows 130 degrees.

4. Remove from the grill, and let rest for 10 minutes.

5. Spoon yellow rice in the center of a plate, and top with black beans.

6. Slice skirt steak and layer slices on top of the black beans.

7. Spoon the plantain salsa around the plate and on top of the steak.

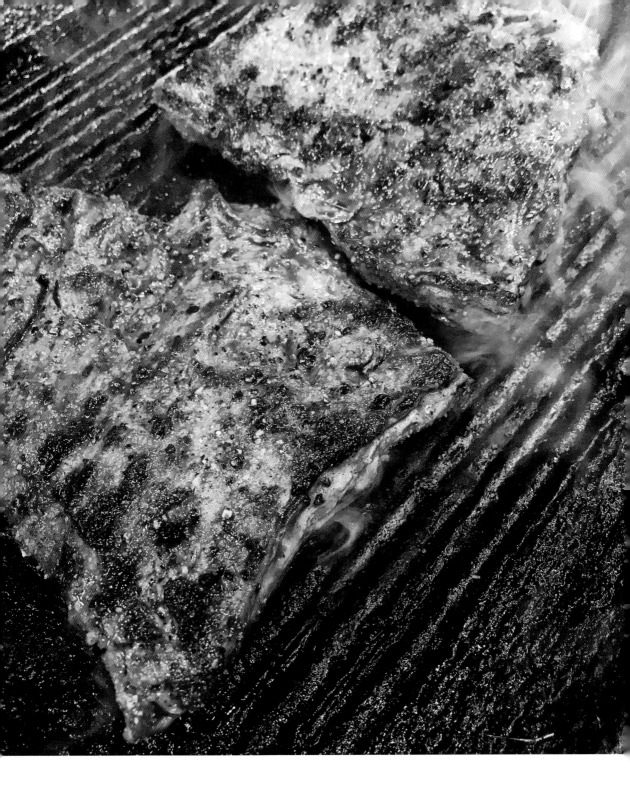

Chicken Parmesan with Cumin-Scented Quinoa

For Chicken Parmesan

4 chicken breasts, fat trimmed and sliced in half

1 cup gluten-free bread crumbs

2 teaspoons oregano

¼ cup grated Parmesan cheese

2 whole eggs beaten

2 tablespoons milk

½ teaspoon Creole seasoning

2 cups tomato sauce

1 pound buffalo mozzarella sliced into 8 pieces

Shredded parmesan cheese

Chopped chives

Cooking spray

For Quinoa

1 cup quinoa

1 tablespoon grape seed oil

1 medium red onion, chopped

2 cloves garlic, minced

2 teaspoons cumin

1 teaspoon smoked paprika

2 cups low-sodium chicken broth

Kosher salt and fresh ground pepper

For Marinara Sauce

2 tablespoons olive oil

1 cup onions, chopped

3 garlic cloves, sliced thin

1 small carrot, diced

2 teaspoons dried thyme

1 teaspoon dried oregano

3 ½ cups canned, fire-roasted tomatoes

Kosher salt fresh ground pepper

Marinara Sauce

1. Sauté onions and carrots in a medium pan over medium heat.

2. Season with salt and pepper, and stir often until onions and carrots are soft.

3. Add garlic, and cook until softened being careful not to burn the mixture.

4. Add thyme and oregano.

5. Stir in roasted tomatoes with juices, and bring to a boil.

6. Reduce heat, and bring to a simmer stirring often to prevent sticking until sauce has thickened.

7. Adjust seasonings, and let sauce cool.

Quinoa

1. Heat 1 tablespoon grape seed oil in a medium saucepan over medium-high heat.

2. Add in red onion, garlic, cumin, and smoked paprika, and stir frequently until softened and fragrant.

3. Add in the chicken broth, and bring to a boil.

4. Stir in quinoa, and reduce to a simmer, cover and cook for 15 minutes. Fluff, and set aside until ready for use.

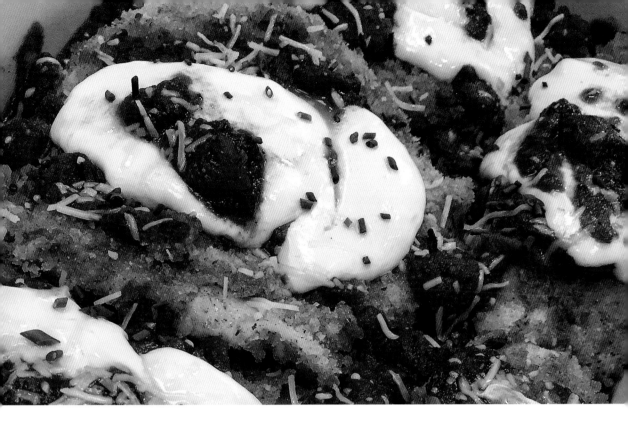

Chicken Parmesan

1. Preheat your oven to 450 degrees. Spray a large baking sheet with cooking spray.

2. Pour ¼ cup of the marinara sauce on the bottom of a casserole dish then top with cooked quinoa.

3. In a large bowl, combine breadcrumbs, oregano, Creole seasoning and parmesan cheese.

4. In another bowl, combine eggs, milk and Creole seasoning.

5. Dip the chicken into the egg mixture, then dip it into the breadcrumb mixture.

6. Place breadcrumb-crusted chicken on the prepared baking sheet, and repeat until all of the chicken has been coated.

7. Lightly spray breaded chicken with more oil on top, and bake until golden brown.

8. Remove chicken from oven, and place on top of the quinoa.

9. Spoon sauce over each piece of chicken, and top each with a slice of mozzarella cheese.

10. Bake until cheese is melted.

11. Garnish with Parmesan cheese and chives.

Herb-Roasted Veal Chop with Farro-Roasted Broccoli and Herb Garlic Butter

For Herb Garlic Butter

¼ cup unsalted butter, room
    temperature

2 teaspoons fresh rosemary, chopped

2 garlic cloves, minced

1 teaspoon Worcestershire sauce

For Veal Chops

Four 1 ½-inch veal chops

2 garlic cloves, minced

2 tablespoons chopped fresh thyme

4 tablespoons extra-virgin olive oil

Kosher salt and fresh ground pepper

½ teaspoon Dijon mustard

1 cup beef broth

For Farro

1 cup farro

2 tablespoons grape seed oil

1 large shallot, diced

2 garlic cloves, sliced

Kosher salt and fresh ground pepper

3 cups low-sodium chicken broth

1 tablespoon fresh thyme

For Roasted Broccoli

1 pound broccoli, rinsed and trimmed

2 tablespoons grape seed oil

2 cloves garlic, minced

Kosher salt and fresh ground pepper

Herb Garlic Butter

1. In a small bowl, combine butter, rosemary, garlic and Worcestershire sauce.

2. Wrap butter in plastic wrap, roll into a log and chill.

Farro

1. Heat one tablespoon of the grape seed oil in a medium saucepan over medium-high heat.

2. Add faro. Cook until fragrant and toasted stirring often for four to five minutes.

3. Remove farro from the saucepan, and add the remaining one tablespoon of grape seed oil.

4. Add in shallots and garlic, and stir frequently until softened.

5. Season with salt and pepper.

6. Return toasted farro to the pan, and stir to coat each grain with seasoned shallots and garlic.

7. Add broth, and bring to a boil.

8. Reduce heat to medium, cover and stir occasionally until liquid is absorbed and farro is tender. This should take 20 to 25 minutes.

9. Stir in fresh thyme, and adjust seasonings.

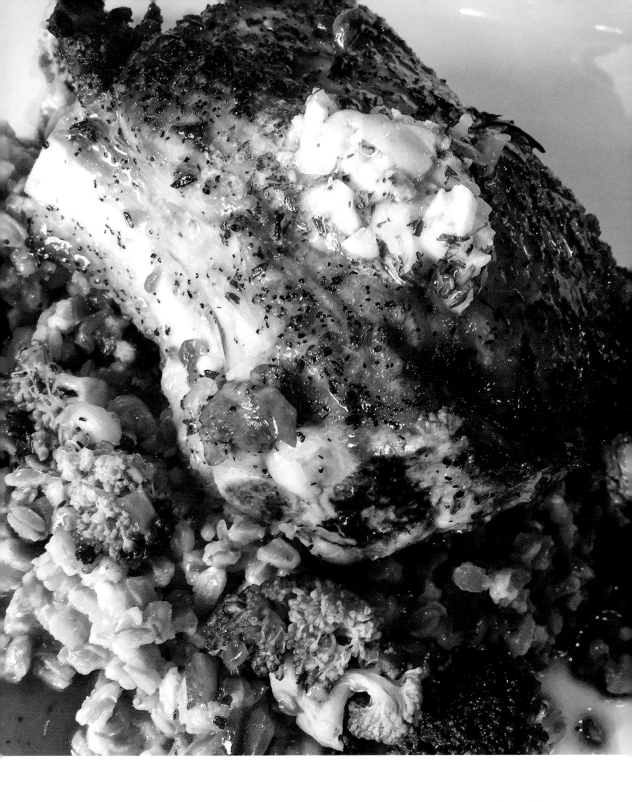

Broccoli

1. Preheat your oven to 400 degrees.

2. Cut your broccoli into bite-size pieces.

3. Toss the broccoli, grape seed oil and garlic together in a medium bowl and season with salt and pepper.

4. Pour broccoli out on to a baking pan, and place in the oven.

5. Roast just until the broccoli is tender, or about eight to 10 more minutes.

Veal Chops

1. Preheat your oven to 400 degrees.

2. In a small bowl, stir together thyme, salt, pepper and olive oil.

3. Rub veal chops with herb mixture.

4. Cover veal chops in plastic wrap, and refrigerate for 30 minutes.

5. Heat remaining olive oil in a large cast-iron skillet over medium-high heat.

6. Brown veal chops about three minutes on each side.

7. Transfer the skillet to the pre-heated oven.

8. Roast veal chops until an instant-read thermometer shows 155 to 160 degrees.

9. Remove veal chops from the pan and keep warm on an oven-proof dish.

10. Pour off fat from skillet.

11. Add Dijon and broth to the skillet, and return to the stove over high heat.

12. Scrape the skillet to dislodge the brown bits stuck to the bottom. This process is called deglazing.

13. Boil the broth until reduced by half.

14. Place one tablespoon of the garlic herb butter on each veal chop, and return to the oven just until the butter starts to melt.

15. Spoon farro into the center of the plate, and top with the butter-coated veal chop.

16. Spoon roasted broccoli around the plate, and finish with the pan sauce.

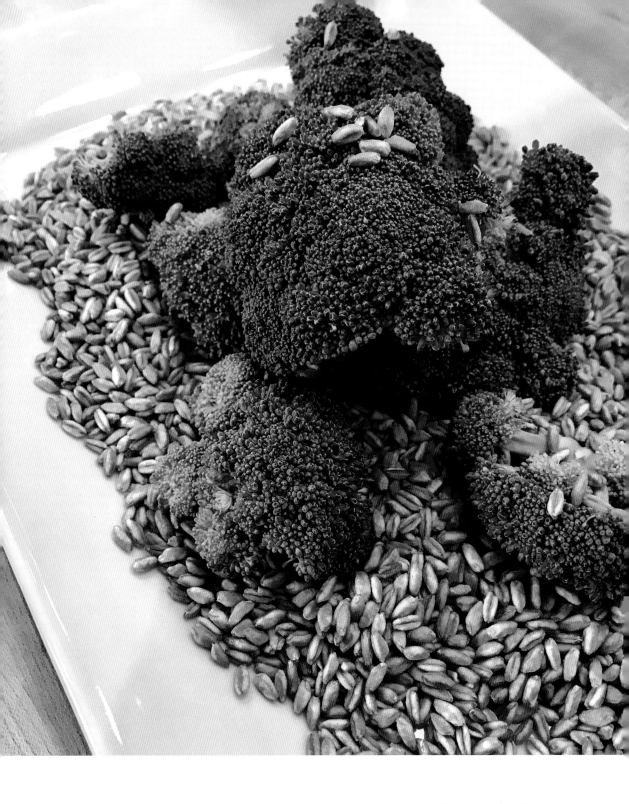

Grilled Bison Filet with Asparagus Fries and Port Jus

For Bison

Four 6-ounce bison filets

½ cup extra-virgin olive oil

¼ cup balsamic vinegar

¼ cup port wine

1 tablespoon stone ground mustard

1 tablespoon honey

2 cloves garlic, minced

2 teaspoons red pepper flakes

1 tablespoon fresh rosemary, chopped

1 tablespoon fresh thyme, chopped

Kosher salt and fresh ground pepper

For Asparagus Fries

1 pound asparagus, trimmed

3 eggs, lightly beaten

½ cup brown rice flour

2 cups gluten-free panko breadcrumbs

2 tablespoons fresh thyme

¼ cup asiago cheese, grated

1 teaspoon Creole seasoning

For Port Jus

1 tablespoon grape seed oil

1 shallot, chopped

1 garlic clove, sliced

¾ cup port

¾ cup red wine

1 sprig rosemary

1 bay leaf

3 cups beef broth

Kosher salt and fresh ground pepper

1 teaspoon unsalted butter

Asparagus Fries

1. Preheat your oven to 425 degrees.

2. Combine panko, thyme, asiago and Creole seasoning in a bowl.

3. Dredge the asparagus in the rice flour, dip in the egg and then dig into the panko mixture.

4. Place the asparagus in a single layer on a wire rack on a baking sheet, and bake until golden brown.

Port Jus

1. In a medium saucepan and over medium-high heat, sauté shallots and garlic in one tablespoon grape seed oil until they start to caramelize.

2. Add port, wine and rosemary.

3. Reduce sauce by half.

4. Add beef broth, and reduce sauce by half.

5. Strain sauce to remove all solids, and return sauce to the stove.

6. Bring sauce to a boil then reduce the temperature, and let simmer for five minutes.

7. Whisk in butter, and adjust seasonings.

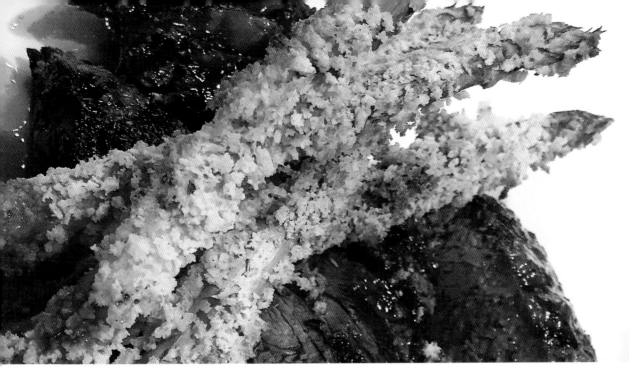

Steaks

1. Combine balsamic vinegar, port, mustard, honey, garlic, red pepper flakes, rosemary and thyme in a medium bowl, and whisk together.

2. While still whisking, drizzle in olive oil in a steady stream until well incorporated.

3. Season marinade with salt and pepper.

4. Place the steaks in a large Ziploc bag, and pour in marinade.

5. Let steaks marinate for about one hour.

6. Prepare a medium-hot fire in a charcoal grill, or heat a gas grill to high.

7. Remove steaks from the marinade, and let them come to room temperature.

8. Grill steaks until cooked to desired doneness, five to six minutes per side for medium rare.

9. Transfer steaks to a plate, and let rest for five minutes.

10. Slice steak and place in the center of the plate, top with asparagus fries and drizzle with port jus. Sprinkle a little salt on sliced steak right before serving.

Mutton Snapper Provençal with Roasted Garlic Cauliflower Puree

For Snapper

Four, 6-ounce filets of mutton snapper

2 tablespoons grape seed oil

Kosher salt and fresh ground pepper

For Provençal Sauce

2 tablespoons extra-virgin olive oil

½ medium red onion, finely sliced

3 cloves of garlic, sliced

1 tablespoon tomato paste

3 cups canned, fire-roasted tomatoes

1 cup white wine

1 bay leaf

¼ teaspoon anchovy paste

½ cup Kalamata olives,
   pitted and halved

2 teaspoons fresh thyme

1 teaspoon fresh basil

Kosher salt and fresh ground pepper

¼ cup green onions, for garnish

For Roasted Garlic Cauliflower Puree

1 head cauliflower, washed with core
   removed and chopped

1 tablespoon grape seed oil

8 cloves garlic, roasted

3 tablespoons unsalted butter

1 cup chicken broth

½ teaspoon cumin

Kosher salt and fresh ground pepper

Provençal Sauce

1. Heat two tablespoons of the olive oil in a medium saucepan over medium-high heat.

2. Add the onion and garlic to the pan, and sauté stirring often until softened but not browned.

3. Add in the tomato paste, and stir to combine.

4. Add the fire-roasted tomatoes, wine, bay leaf, anchovy paste and olives.

5. Cook over medium heat stirring occasionally until the sauce has thickened

6. Discard the bay leaf, and adjust seasonings.

7. Heat the remaining ¼ cup of olive oil in a small saucepan.

8. Add the garlic and cook over moderately-low heat stirring until golden brown. This usually takes about five minutes.

9. Add the olives and capers, and cook until heated through. It should take three to five minutes.

10. Add the mixture to the tomato sauce along with the chopped herbs, and season with pepper.

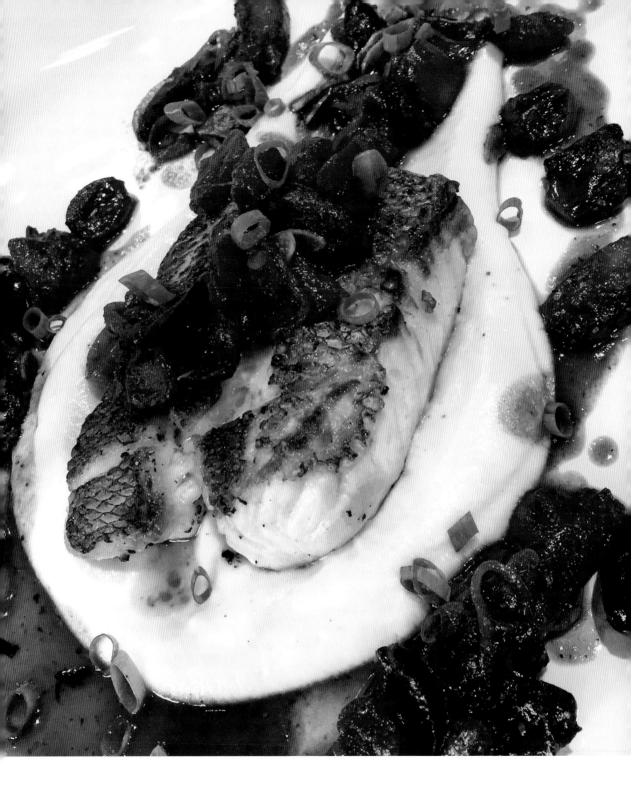

Roasted Garlic Cauliflower Puree

1. Preheat your oven to 350 degrees.

2. Place garlic cloves on a sheet of foil paper and drizzle with grape seed oil.

3. Season with salt and pepper, and loosely wrap in foil.

4. Roast garlic for about 15 minutes or until the cloves start to turn light brown and translucent.

5. Remove garlic from the oven, and set aside until ready for use.

6. Combine cauliflower and chicken broth in a medium pot over high heat, and bring to a boil.

7. Reduce the heat to low, and cover the pot.

8. Let the cauliflower steep until soft. This should take 10 to 15 minutes.

9. Strain the cauliflower, and combine it with the garlic, butter and cumin in the bowl of a food processor or blender. Don't throw away the broth.

10. Blend the cauliflower until light and smooth. If it's not smooth enough, carefully add in broth to achieve the desired texture.

11. Season with salt and pepper.

Snapper

1. Preheat your oven to 400 degrees.

2. Score the skin of each filet to prevent it from curling during cooking.

3. Season each filet on both sides with salt and pepper.

4. Heat two tablespoons of grape seed oil in a cast-iron skillet over medium-high heat.

5. Place each snapper filet down in the pan (skin side down), and cook until skin starts to brown. This should take about two minutes. Resist the temptation to keep checking to see if the skin is browned. When it releases from the pan, it's ready.

6. Turn the snapper, and place the skillet in oven. Roast for another seven minutes.

7. Remove snapper from the oven.

8. Spoon cauliflower puree in the center of a plate, and run the spoon through it from left to right to create a well.

9. Place a piece of the roasted snapper in the well of the cauliflower.

10. Spoon Provençal sauce over the snapper and around the puree.

11. Garnish with green onions.

Chef's Tip:

Always taste as you go. It's the only way to know if you're doing it right.

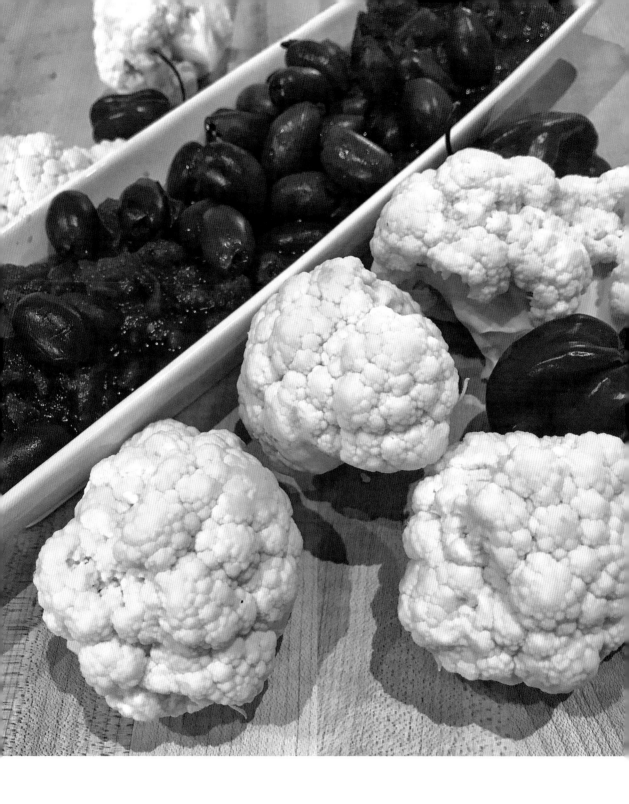

Turkey and Spinach Meatballs

For Meatballs

Nonstick, vegetable oil spray

1 tablespoon grape seed oil

3 cups spinach, raw

2 garlic cloves, minced

¼ small, red onion, finely chopped

1 large egg, beaten

1 pound lean ground turkey

½ pound ground turkey thigh meat

½ cup asiago cheese, finely grated

½ cup old-fashioned oats

1½ tablespoons fresh thyme

2 teaspoons curry powder

1 ½ teaspoons Creole seasoning

1 tablespoon Dijon mustard

Kosher salt and fresh ground pepper

For Coconut Curry Sauce

2 tablespoons coconut oil

1 medium yellow onion, finely chopped

4 cloves garlic, minced

1½ teaspoons fresh ginger, minced

½ scotch bonnet, minced (jalapeño
   pepper can be substituted)

3 ½ tablespoons Jamaican curry powder

1 cup low-sodium chicken broth

2 cups coconut milk

4 sprigs fresh thyme

1 bay leaf

Kosher salt and freshly ground
   black pepper

Coconut Curry Sauce

1. Heat the coconut oil in a medium saucepan over medium heat.

2. Add the onions, garlic, ginger and scotch bonnet pepper, and stir until the onions have softened.

3. Add curry powder, and continue to cook until curry powder turns deep golden brown.

4. Add the chicken broth, coconut milk, thyme and bay leaf.

5. Reduce heat to low and simmer until sauce is lightly reduced.

6. Adjust seasonings with salt and pepper.

7. Add turkey meatballs to coconut curry sauce, and continue to simmer until meatballs are heated through.

Turkey and Spinach Meatballs

1. Preheat your oven to 400 degrees.

2. Line a baking sheet with foil, and spray with non-stick spray.

3. Heat grape seed oil in a large sauté pan over medium-high heat.

4. Add garlic and onions, and stir frequently until fragrant.

5. Add spinach, and season with salt and pepper.

6. Cook spinach until it begins to wilt.

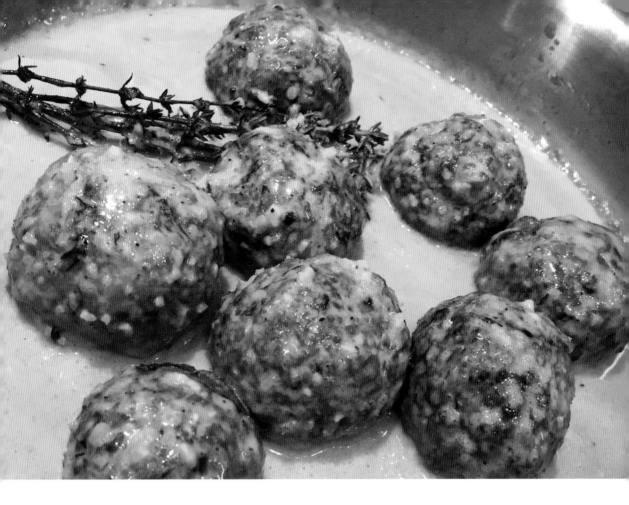

7. Transfer spinach to a clean plate, and let it cool.

8. Once cooled, squeeze spinach in paper towels to remove excess moisture then chop.

9. Combine chopped spinach, egg, turkey, asiago cheese, oats, thyme, curry powder, Creole seasoning and mustard in a large mixing bowl.

10. Mix ingredients together until well incorporated.

11. Form mixture into balls and place on the foil-lined baking sheet. If you wet your hands a little, it'll make it easier to form the mix into balls.

12. Bake meatballs in preheated oven until browned.

13. Remove from the oven, and simmer in coconut curry sauce.

Kale and Peach Caesar Salad with Roasted Salmon Nuggets and Cilantro Caesar Dressing

For Kale and Peach Salad

2 bunches curly kale, tough stems
    removed, leaves roughly chopped

½ medium red onion, sliced thin

4 large ripe peaches, cut into
    ½-inch wedges

For salmon

Two, 6-ounce salmon fillets, cut into
    2-inch pieces

2 teaspoons Creole seasoning

Grape seed oil cooking spray

For Cilantro Caesar Dressing

¼ cup fresh lime juice

8 anchovy fillets packed in oil, drained

2 garlic cloves

1 teaspoon Dijon mustard

1 tablespoon honey

¾ cup extra-virgin olive oil

1 bunch cilantro, rinsed and patted dry

½ cup finely grated Parmesan

Kosher salt and freshly ground
    black pepper

Salmon

1. Season salmon with Creole seasoning.

2. Coat a medium nonstick sauté pan with cooking spray over medium-high heat.

3. Cook salmon until it's golden brown and opaque.

4. Remove from heat, and reserve until ready for use.

Cilantro Caesar Dressing

1. Combine lime juice, anchovy, garlic, mustard and honey in a blender, and purée until smooth.

2. With the motor running, drizzle oil in a slow steady stream until all of the oil has been incorporated.

3. Add in the cilantro, and puree until fully blended.

4. Pour dressing into a medium bowl, and stir in ¼ cup Parmesan cheese.

5. Adjust seasoning with salt and pepper.

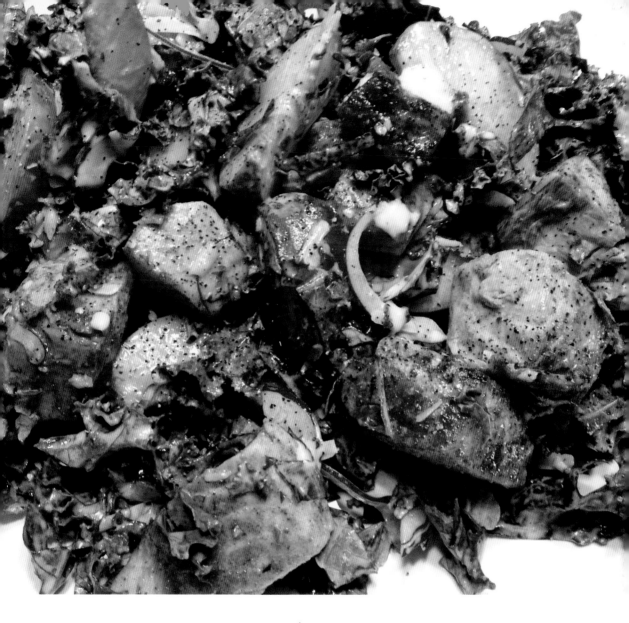

Kale and Peach Caesar Salad

1. Light a grill, or preheat a grill pan.

2. Brush the peaches with olive oil, and grill over high heat until tender. Transfer to a plate until ready for use.

3. In a large bowl, combine kale, onions, peaches, salmon nuggets and dressing.

4. Toss until well coated.

5. Garnish with remaining cheese.

Rosemary and Balsamic-Roasted Yard Bird with Truffled Fingerling Potatoes

For Chicken

1 whole chicken, split and
    breast bones removed

4 teaspoons extra-virgin olive oil

3 garlic cloves, minced

2 tablespoons Dijon mustard

4 teaspoons fresh, chopped rosemary

Kosher salt and fresh ground pepper

¼ cup low-fat balsamic dressing

For Truffled Fingerling Potatoes

2 pounds fingerling potatoes, scrubbed,
    patted dry and halved

2 tablespoons olive oil

1 tablespoon minced garlic

 Kosher salt freshly ground pepper

1 tablespoon white truffle oil

2 tablespoons grated Parmesan cheese

Fingerling Potatoes

1. Place potatoes on a foil-lined baking sheet.

2. Drizzle with olive oil, and season with salt and pepper.

3. Toss well to combine.

4. Bake until potatoes are browned and tender.

5. Remove from the oven, and toss with Parmesan cheese and truffle oil.

6. Transfer potatoes to a large oven-proof baking dish.

Chicken

1. Preheat your oven to 400 degrees.

2. Line a baking sheet with foil, and top with a rack.

3. Place each half of chicken skin side down on the rack.

4. Drizzle one teaspoon of the olive oil over each half of the chicken, and rub it in to distribute it evenly.

5. Spread one tablespoon of the mustard over each half of the chicken.

6. Sprinkle minced garlic on both chicken halves.

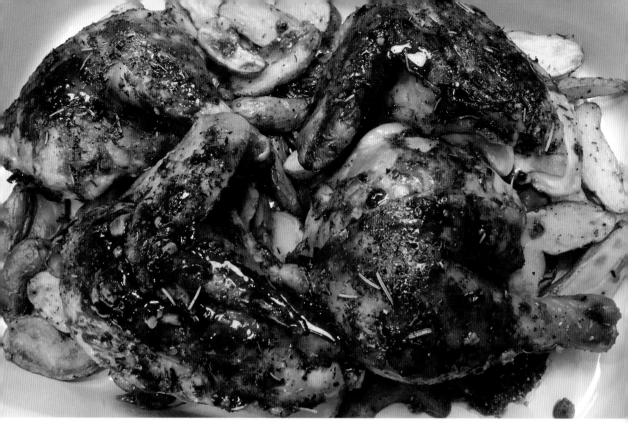

7. Sprinkle one teaspoon of the rosemary on each half of the chicken.

8. Season with salt and pepper.

9. Turn chicken halves over so the skin side is up.

10. Drizzle one teaspoon of the olive oil over each half of the chicken, and rub it in to distribute it evenly.

11. Season with salt and pepper.

12. Sprinkle one teaspoon of the rosemary on each half of the chicken.

13. Transfer chicken to the oven, and cook about 20-30 minutes, or until the internal temperature reads 165 on an instant-read thermometer.

14. Place chicken skin side up on top of fingerling potatoes in the large baking dish.

15. Drizzle balsamic dressing over the chicken.

16. Tent baking dish with foil, and place in the pre-heated oven.

17. Cook for an additional 10 minutes.

18. Remove foil, and serve.

Stewed Okra and Tomatoes with Shrimp

1 pound fresh okra, tops
    trimmed and split

2 cups canned, fire-roasted tomatoes

3 tablespoons extra-virgin olive oil

1 pound jumbo shrimp,
    peeled and deveined

2 teaspoons Creole seasoning

1 teaspoon smoked paprika

½ medium yellow onion, sliced thin

1 green bell pepper, diced

¼ cup celery, diced

2 cloves garlic, minced

Kosher salt and fresh ground pepper

2 teaspoons fresh thyme

½ teaspoon cayenne pepper

½ cup low-sodium chicken broth

1. Combine shrimp, Creole seasoning and smoked paprika in a medium bowl and toss to combine.

2. Heat one tablespoon of the olive oil in a large cast-iron skillet over medium- high heat.

3. Add seasoned shrimp to the skillet, and cook until just opaque.

4. Transfer shrimp to a bowl, and set aside until ready for use. Don't clean the skillet.

5. Add one tablespoon of the olive oil to the skillet over medium-high heat.

6. Cook okra stirring frequently, and season with salt and pepper.

7. Remove okra from the skillet just as it begins to soften, and set aside.

8. Add remaining oil to the skillet.

9. Add the onions, celery and bell pepper.

10. Cook until onions, celery and bell peppers are lightly browned.

11. Stir in the garlic. Add the tomatoes, cayenne and thyme while stirring occasionally.

12. Pour in the chicken broth, and stir to combine.

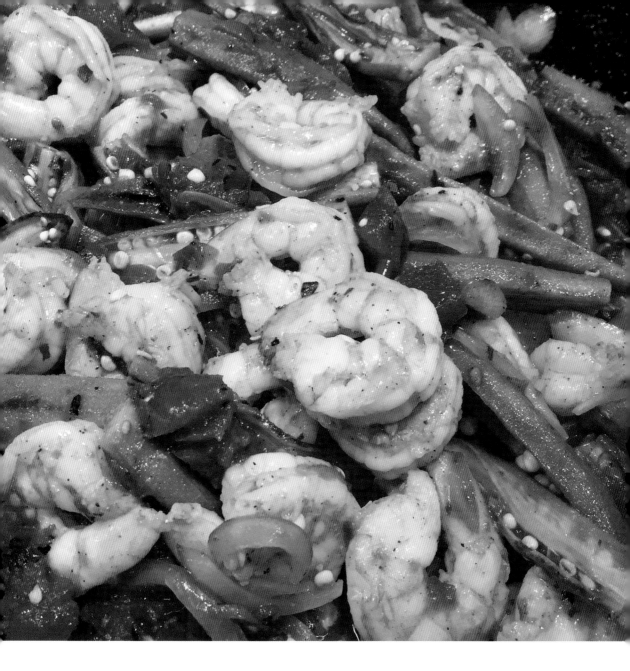

13. Reduce the heat, and simmer covered for 15 to 20 minutes.

14. Remove the cover, and fold in reserved shrimp and okra.

15. Adjust the seasonings, and cook until shrimp and okra are warmed through.

16. Serve alone or over your favorite grain.

Jumbo Lump Crab Cakes over Heirloom Tomato and Quinoa Salad with Lemon Honey Vinaigrette

For Crab Cakes

- 1 egg, beaten
- ¼ cup avocado mayonnaise
- ¼ teaspoon cayenne pepper
- 1 teaspoon smoked paprika
- ½ teaspoon cumin
- 1 teaspoon Creole seasoning
- 1 pound jumbo lump crabmeat, drained and picked
- 1 tablespoon fresh cilantro, finally chopped
- Grape seed oil for frying

For Tomato and Quinoa Salad

- 1 cup cooked quinoa
- 1 English cucumber, quartered and sliced
- 1 medium red onion, sliced thin
- 2 pounds large heirloom tomatoes, cut into ½-inch wedges
- Microgreens for garnish

For Lemon Honey Vinaigrette

- ½ cup olive oil
- ¼ cup fresh lemon juice
- ¼ teaspoon cayenne pepper
- 1 tablespoon shallot, minced
- 3 teaspoons Dijon mustard
- 1 teaspoon lemon zest
- 2 tablespoons honey
- Kosher salt and fresh ground pepper

Crab Cakes

1. Combine egg, mayonnaise, cayenne, paprika, cumin and Creole seasoning in a medium mixing bowl.

2. Mix thoroughly to fully incorporate flavors.

3. In a separate bowl, combine crabmeat and cilantro.

4. Add wet mix to crab mixture, and fold in.

5. Portion crab mix into patties and refrigerate at least 15 minutes to help set.

6. Heat oil in a medium, cast-iron skillet over medium heat.

7. Cook patties until golden brown on both sides. This should take about two minutes per side.

8. Drain on a paper towel lined pan.

Lemon Honey Vinaigrette

1. Whisk together the lemon juice, pepper, shallots, mustard, zest and honey in a medium mixing bowl until well blended.

2. Whisk in oil in a slow stream until the dressing is well blended.

3. Season with salt and pepper.

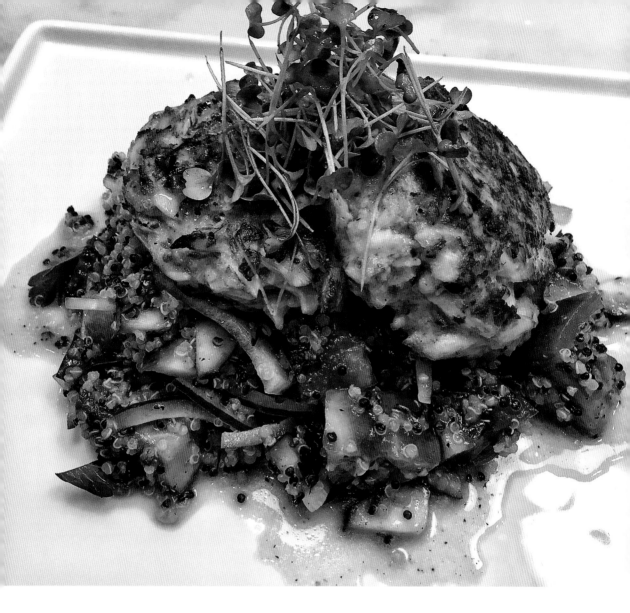

Tomato and Quinoa Salad

1. Combine quinoa, cucumbers, onions and tomatoes in a large bowl.

2. Gently toss salad with lemon honey vinaigrette.

3. Spoon salad in the center of the plate.

4. Top with two of the crab cakes.

5. Garnish with microgreens.

6. Drizzle lemon honey vinaigrette over the top of microgreens and around plate.

Jumbo Lump Crab Coleslaw

Juice of 1 lime

1 garlic clove, minced

1 tablespoon ginger, minced

2 teaspoons ponzu

1 teaspoon sambal

1 teaspoon sesame oil

2 tablespoons honey

¼ cup avocado mayonnaise

1 ½ teaspoons rice vinegar

Kosher salt and fresh ground pepper

1/3 cup cilantro, chopped

2 scallions, chopped

2 cups purple cabbage, shredded

1 red bell pepper, sliced thin

2 cups jumbo lump crabmeat, drained and picked

1 cup mandarin oranges, drained

1. In a medium bowl, whisk together the lime juice, garlic, ginger, Ponzu, sambal, sesame oil, honey, mayonnaise and rice vinegar until well incorporated.

2. Taste, and season with salt and pepper.

3. In a separate bowl, combine Cilantro, scallions, cabbage, bell pepper, crab, and oranges.

4. Fold in coleslaw dressing, adjust seasonings and serve.

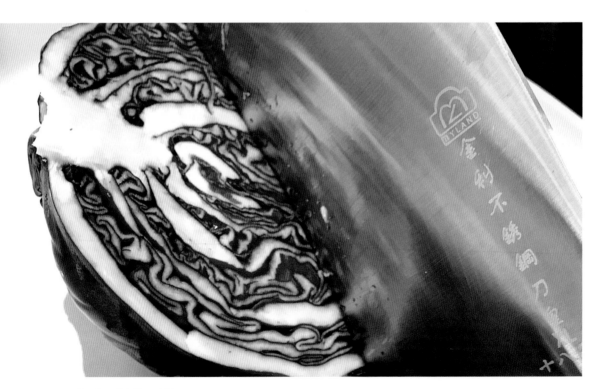

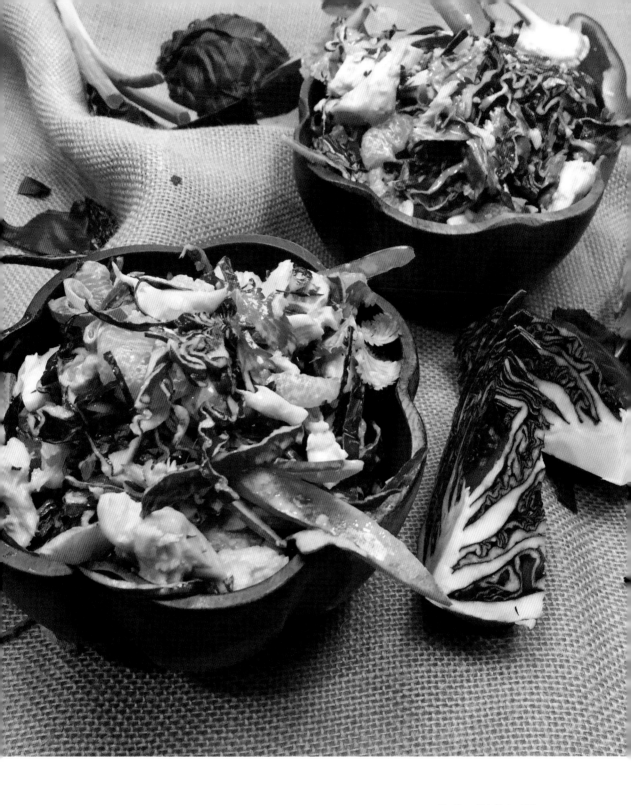

Stewed Chicken Thighs with Garbanzo Beans

8 skin-on, bone-in chicken thighs,
  trimmed of excess fat

2 cans garbanzo beans, drained

1 ½ tablespoons grape seed oil

2 tablespoons Creole seasoning

1 small yellow onion, diced

1 rib celery, diced

3 cloves garlic, minced

1 red bell pepper, diced

2 jalapeño peppers, seeded
  and chopped

2 tablespoons tomato paste

1 bay leaf

3 sprigs fresh thyme, tied with butchers
  twine

½ cup low-sodium chicken broth

Kosher salt and freshly ground
  black pepper

1. Preheat your oven to 425 degrees.

2. Heat oil in a large cast-iron skillet over medium-high heat.

3. Season chicken thighs evenly with Creole seasoning.

4. Cook chicken thighs skin side down until skin is browned and crispy being careful not to overcrowd the pan.

5. Turn thighs over, and continue cooking until browned.

6. Remove the browned thighs from the pan, and pour off all the oil from the skillet. Do not clean the skillet.

7. Return the skillet to the stove, and add the remaining ½ tablespoon of the grape seed oil.

8. Add onion, celery, garlic, bell pepper and jalapeño, and cook until vegetables soften.

9. Add tomato paste, and stir until it begins to darken.

10. Add garbanzo beans, broth, thyme and bay leaf, and bring to a simmer.

11. Adjust seasonings with salt and pepper.

12. Return browned thighs to the skillet skin side up.

13. Cover skillet with and place in the pre-heated oven.

14. Cook for about 20 minutes or until thighs are done.

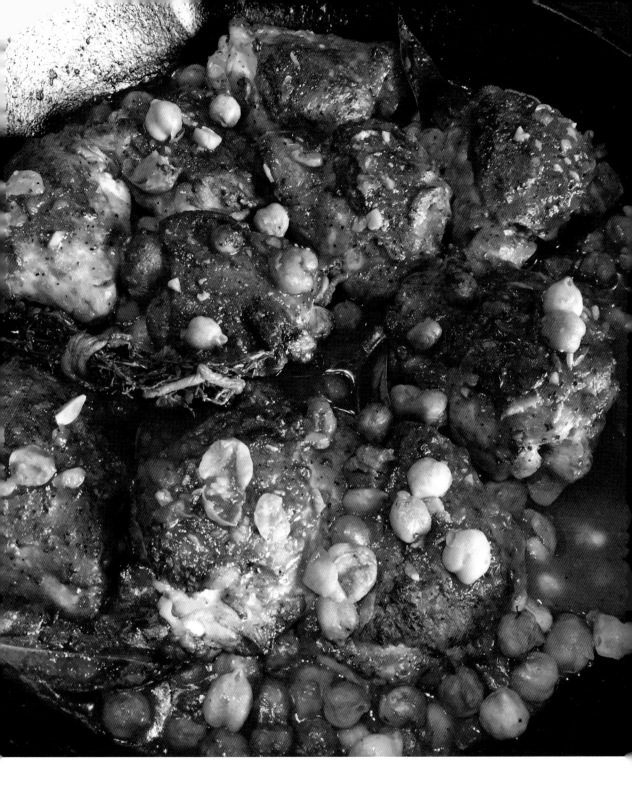

Shepherd's Pie with Creamy Golden Cauliflower and Smoked Gouda Crust

For Pie Filling

2 tablespoons grape seed oil

2 pounds ground bison

1 cup red onion, chopped

3 cloves garlic, minced

2 medium carrots, cut into rounds

1 rib celery, minced

1 bay leaf

2 tablespoons chopped fresh thyme

2 tablespoons tomato paste

1 ½ cups low-sodium beef broth

1 cup frozen peas, thawed

Kosher salt and fresh ground pepper

For Cauliflower Topping

2 small heads golden cauliflower,
   cut into florets

3 garlic cloves

2 tablespoons butter

Kosher salt and fresh ground pepper

4 ounces grated, smoked gouda cheese

Pie Filling

1. Heat grape seed oil in a large cast-iron skillet over medium-high heat.

2. Brown the ground bison until cooked through.

3. Transfer the bison to a medium bowl using a slotted spoon, and reserve.

4. Drain all but one tablespoon of the drippings from the skillet.

5. Return the skillet to heat and add onion, garlic, carrots and celery, and cook until vegetables have softened.

6. Return ground bison to the skillet with the bay leaf and thyme.

7. Stir in tomato paste, and cook until fragrant.

8. Stir in broth and peas, and season with salt and pepper.

9. Stir until sauce thickens.

10. Remove the filling from heat, and transfer to a large casserole dish.

Cauliflower Topping

1. Preheat your oven to 400 degrees.

2. Steam cauliflower and garlic in a steaming basket set in a large stockpot of boiling water.

3. Cover and steam until cauliflower is very tender.

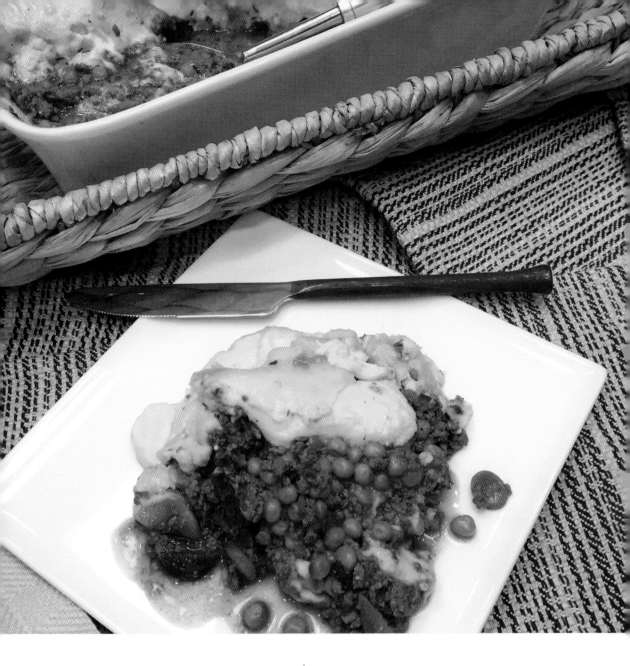

4. Transfer cauliflower, garlic and butter to a blender or food processor and puree until smooth.

5. Adjust seasonings with salt and pepper

6. Spread cauliflower puree over the bison filling, and sprinkle with smoked gouda cheese.

7. Bake until filling is bubbling and cheese is melted.

Roasted Mussels in Spicy Coconut Broth

2 tablespoons coconut oil

2 shallots, chopped

3 teaspoons fresh ginger, minced

4 garlic cloves, sliced

2 red chili peppers,
de-seeded and chopped

1 can coconut milk

2 tablespoons fish sauce

1 tablespoon coconut sugar

Juice of 2 limes

¼ cup cilantro, chopped

3 pounds mussels,
scrubbed and de-bearded

1. Heat the coconut oil in a large pot over medium-high heat.

2. Add the shallots, and sauté until translucent.

3. Add the ginger, garlic and peppers, and stir until fragrant.

4. Stir in the coconut milk, fish sauce, sugar and lime juice.

5. Stir using a wooden spoon to scrape up any browned bits that have stuck to the bottom of the pot.

6. Bring the coconut broth to a boil, and cook for about two minutes.

7. Add the mussels and cilantro to the pot and stir to coat them with the liquid.

8. Cover and cook until all the shells have opened.

9. Discard any mussels that remain closed.

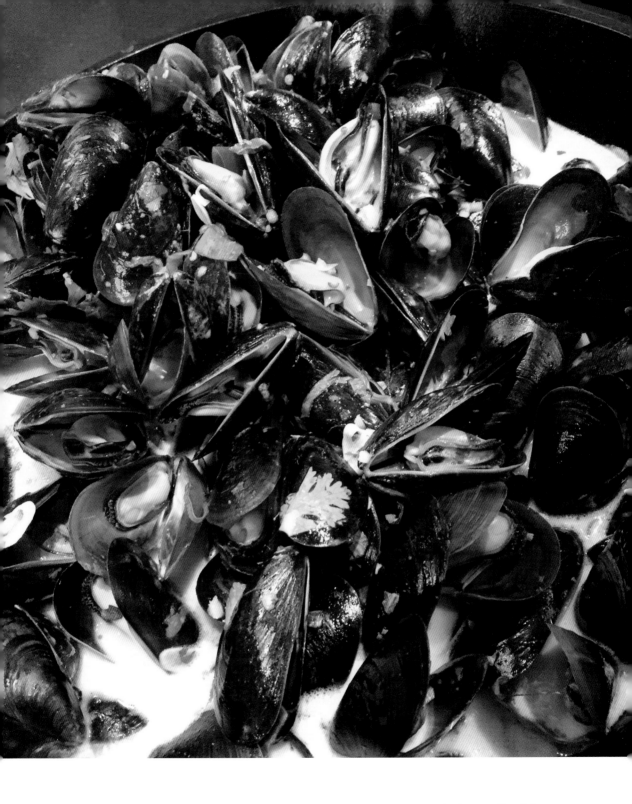

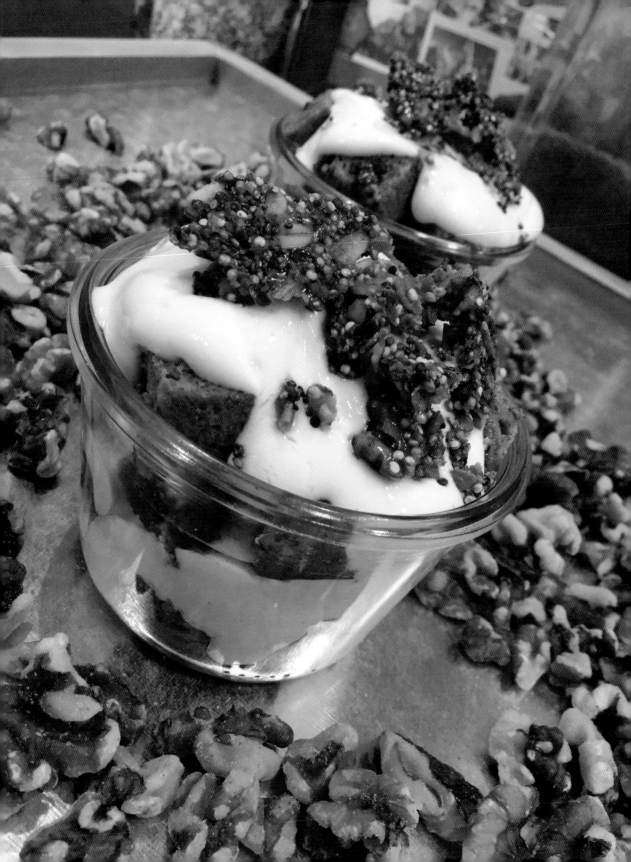

Why Eat Dessert?

I remember as a kid rushing through any meal that had dessert at the end. I didn't matter if it was a slice of my mother's warm rum cake with that wonderful caramelized pecan crust and a single scoop of vanilla ice cream on top that soaked into the pores of the cake like a sponge or my grandmother's simple fruit cocktail strawberry Jell-O delight (the word delight makes it taste extra special, just in case you didn't know) that she'd give me after one of her famous tuna sandwiches. Dessert time was always a happy time.

As of late, desserts have become the bad guy of the meal. It's looked at as cheating if you indulge in having your favorite dessert. This is not the case. Eating desserts as well as other pleasurable foods make your brain release endorphins to elevate your mood. The key, as it is with everything, is to not over do it. There are ways to make desserts a little healthier like substituting granulated sugar for maple syrup (¾ cup maple syrup = 1cup granulated sugar), watching the types of oil you use or something as simple as adding ground flax seeds to cookie dough for added fiber.

In this chapter, you'll see where I've made healthier choices like using yogurt instead of cream cheese in the carrot cake trifle. But I went all out in the chocolate chip cookie and bacon red velvet waffles. Sometimes you want what you want, and there's nothing wrong with that! Life is too short to skip dessert.

Eating Dessert to Win

If you choose to indulge in a dessert, plan it out first. Cut your carbs during dinner and increase your vegetable intake so that you can enjoy your dessert with less guilt.

Flourless Chocolate Cake with Raspberry Sauce

For Cake

- 1 stick unsalted butter
- 2 tablespoons unsalted butter softened (for greasing ramekins)
- ¼ cup maple syrup
- 1 cup semisweet chocolate, chopped
- 3 tablespoons Kahlúa
- 4 eggs
- ½ teaspoon pure, vanilla extract
- ¼ teaspoon kosher salt

For Raspberry Sauce

- ½ cup coconut sugar
- 3 tablespoons water
- 1 pound fresh raspberries
- 1 teaspoon Grand Marnier

Raspberry Sauce

1. Heat the sugar and water in a small saucepan over medium heat stirring until the sugar dissolves completely.

2. Put the raspberries and the syrup in a blender, and puree until smooth.

3. Strain your sauce through a fine mesh sieve to remove the seeds.

4. Whisk in the Grand Marnier.

5. Refrigerate until ready to serve.

Cake

1. Preheat oven to 325 degrees.

2. Grease six oval ramekins with two tablespoons of softened butter.

3. Place the ramekins in a large baking pan, and set to the side.

4. Combine the chocolate, one stick of unsalted butter and Kahlúa in a metal bowl, and melt over a water bath while stirring repeatedly. Once the chocolate is melted, remove the bowl from the heat and set to the side until ready for use.

5. Combine the eggs, maple syrup, vanilla and salt in the bowl of an electric mixer fitted with the whip attachment, and whip until frothy and doubled in size.

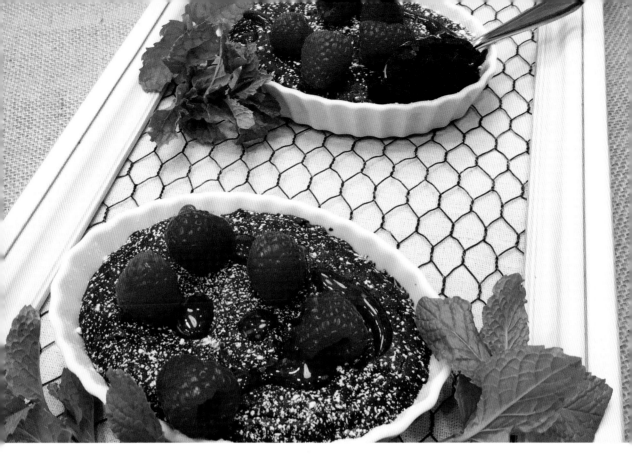

6. Gradually fold in some of the egg mixture into the chocolate mixture with a rubber spatula. Be gentle. The last thing you want to do is to take out all of the air in your egg mixture. The air is what will make you cake nice and light.

7. Continue this process until all of the egg mixture has been folded into the chocolate.

8. Divide the batter between the ramekins, and add enough boiling water to the baking pan to come halfway up the sides of each ramekin.

9. Bake until the cakes have risen and the sides are slightly pulling away.

10. Remove the ramekins from the baking pan, and cool.

11. Serve the cakes in the ramekins with fresh raspberries and a drizzle of raspberry sauce.

Burnt Orange and Butternut Squash Crème Brûlée

For Squash

    1 medium butternut squash, halved lengthwise and seeded

    2 tablespoons unsalted butter

    1 teaspoon cinnamon

    1 teaspoon nutmeg

    1 teaspoon ginger

    2 tablespoons maple syrup

    2 tablespoons orange mango juice

    2 teaspoons kosher salt

For Crème Brûlée

    2 cups roasted butternut squash

    Zest of 2 oranges divided

    $2/3$ cup maple syrup

    5 egg yolks

    2 teaspoons pure vanilla extract

    1 teaspoon cinnamon

    1/4 teaspoon nutmeg

    1/4 teaspoon ginger

    1/4 teaspoon salt

    3 cups heavy cream

    5 tablespoons sugar in the raw

Squash

1. Place squash cut side up on a foil-lined baking sheet.

2. Score each squash in a diamond pattern to ensure the flavor penetrates into the flesh of the squash.

3. Place one tablespoon of butter in the middle of each squash.

4. Drizzle syrup over both halves of the squash.

5. Sprinkle cinnamon, nutmeg, salt and ginger over the flesh of the squash.

6. Finish by pouring one tablespoon of the orange mango juice into the center of the squash.

7. Roast the squash for 45 to 50 minutes, or until it's caramelized and tender. Remove from the oven, and let cool.

Crème Brûlée

1. Preheat oven to 325 degrees.

2. Scoop out the flesh of the butternut squash, and puree that with its juices and the zest of one orange in a blender or food processor until smooth. If you don't have a zester, you can take a sharp knife and carefully slice away the orange peel. You'll want to be careful not to include the white pith because that part is bitter. Once you've removed the peel, you can chop it up finely, and that will be your zest.

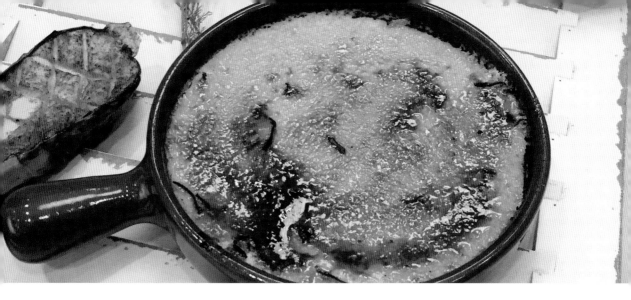

3. Combine two cups of puree and syrup in a large bowl.

4. Add in egg yolks, spices, salt and vanilla to puree, and whisk well to incorporate.

5. Using a medium saucepan, bring your cream to a boil then slowly whisk the hot cream into the squash puree.

6. Strain the mixture into a clean medium bowl to remove all solids.

7. Pour custard into ramekins, and place into a deep roasting pan. Pour boiling water into the pan until it comes halfway up the sides of the ramekins.

8. Bake for 15 minutes, or until the edges are set and the center moves slightly when shaken.

9. Remove the ramekins from the roasting pan, and cool at room temperature for one hour.

10. Cover and refrigerate for at least two hours before serving.

11. Combine the remaining orange zest with five tablespoons of sugar in a small mixing bowl.

12. Using your fingers, grind the zest into the sugar. This will release the orange oils into the sugar.

13. Sprinkle the orange sugar over the top of the custard.

14. Heat the sugar with a kitchen torch until melted and caramelized. The orange zest will get charred during this process. Not to worry, the slight char gives this dessert a delightful smoky finish. If you don't have a kitchen torch, you can use your broiler. Follow the same steps and pass it under your broiler for three minutes, but be careful and watch it closely. It's very easy to scorch the sugar.

Farrow Pudding with Beet Chips and Rum Raisins

For Pudding

1 cup cooked farrow

½ cup raisins

1/3 cup dark rum

¾ cup coconut milk

3 tablespoons maple syrup

1 teaspoon cinnamon

½ teaspoon nutmeg

¼ teaspoon vanilla extract

¼ cup toasted walnuts, chopped

pinch of salt

For Beet Chips

2 golden beets

1 cup water

½ cup sugar

Beets

1. Preheat your oven to 250 degrees.

2. Slice the beets thinly using a mandoline slicer. Please be careful while using the mandoline. It's very easy to cut yourself as you get closer to the end of the beets. If you don't have a mandolin, your sharpest knife will work just as well. But, be warned, you may not have the same consistency throughout your slices.

3. Bring water and sugar to a boil in a small saucepan stirring constantly until sugar dissolves.

4. Add your beets, and reduce the heat to a simmer. Cook until slightly translucent.

5. Using a slotted spoon, transfer beets in a single layer to a baking sheet lined with a nonstick baking mat.

6. Bake for about one hour until dry and slightly firm.

Pudding

1. Combine raisins and rum in a small bowl and cover. Leave raisins to soak for about two hours then drain and place to the side until ready for use.

2. In a medium saucepan, combine cooked farrow, rum raisins (save a few for garnish), coconut milk, maple syrup, cinnamon, nutmeg, vanilla, walnuts and salt.

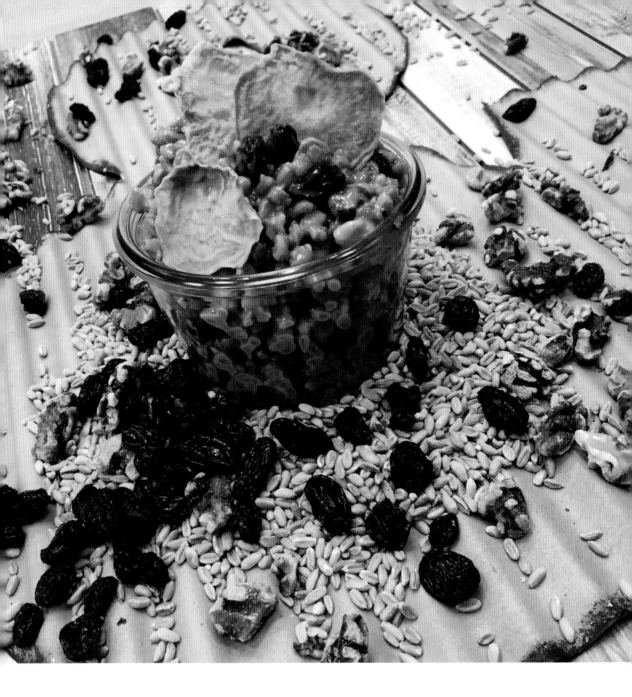

3. Stir over medium heat until warmed throughout and flavors are well incorporated.

4. Adjust you seasonings.

5. To finish, spoon pudding into a bowl, top with beet chips and the extra rum raisins.

Toffee Black Bean Brownies

Non-stick cooking spray

1 cup canned black beans

½ cup canola oil

2 eggs

½ cup Hershey's special dark
   unsweetened cocoa powder

⅔ cup maple syrup

1 teaspoon instant espresso

1 ½ teaspoons vanilla extract

¼ cup chocolate chips

¼ cup bitter sweet chocolate bar pieces

1/3 cup whole wheat flour

½ teaspoon baking powder

½ teaspoon salt

½ toffee pieces

1. Preheat your oven to 350 degrees

2. Grease a 9-by-9 inch square, baking pan.

3. Using a blender or food processor, puree the beans with the canola oil.

4. Add the eggs, special dark cocoa, maple syrup, espresso and vanilla.

5. Melt the chocolate chips, and add to the blender or food processor.

6. Blend on medium high until smooth.

7. In a small bowl, whisk together the flour, baking powder and salt.

8. Add the flour mixture to the blender/food processor and pulse until just incorporated.

9. Stir in the chocolate pieces, and pour the brownie mixture into your prepared pan.

10. Top the brownie mixture with the toffee. You can take a toothpick and swirl the toffee into the brownies if you like.

11. Bake for 20 minutes, or until the surface looks dull around the edges and a toothpick inserted in the middle comes out with just a few crumbs.

12. Let brownies cool for at least 10 minutes before cutting and removing from the pan. I know it's going to be hard to wait, but trust me it's worth it.

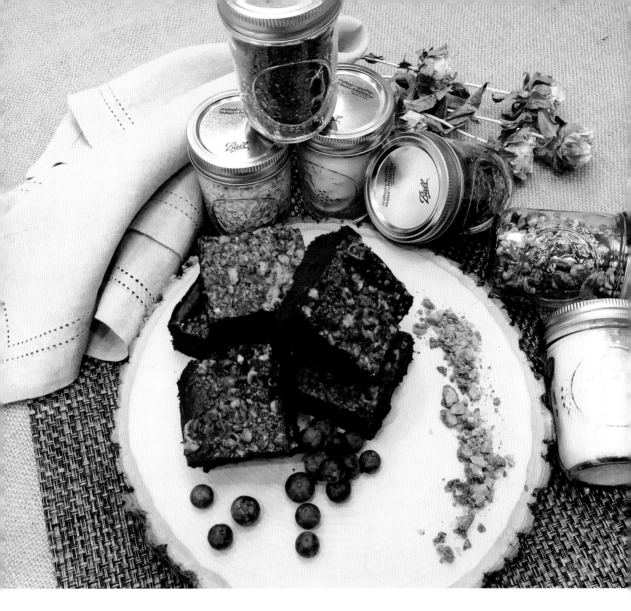

Chef's Note:

One thing that I've tried to do with my clients is to give them foods that they were used to but a little healthier. I had a client that challenged me all the time to see if I could make a healthier version of the items he'd pick. One day he called me up and really wanted me to make him a dessert that he wouldn't feel guilty about eating, and it just so happens that he loved chocolate. So, I made him these brownies (without the toffee) and they were a hit! With or without the toffee, I'm sure you will enjoy them.

Carrot Cake Trifle with Walnut Quinoa Brittle

For Cake

5 large eggs

1 ½ cups maple syrup

2 cups coconut oil, melted

2 tablespoons mango orange juice

1 ½ tablespoons bourbon

1 ½ teaspoons vanilla extract

4 cups whole wheat flour

4 cups grated rainbow carrots

1 cup crushed pineapple

1 cup raisins

2 ½ teaspoons baking soda

½ teaspoon baking powder

1 ½ teaspoons salt

2 teaspoons ground cinnamon

½ teaspoon ground ginger

½ teaspoon 5 spice

1 teaspoon ground nutmeg

Six, 8-ounce Mason jars

For Brittle

1 cup uncooked rainbow quinoa

1 ½ cups walnuts, chopped

½ cup rolled oats

4 tablespoons chia seeds

4 tablespoons coconut sugar

4 tablespoons walnut oil

1 cup maple syrup

For Frosting

2 cups vanilla Greek yogurt

2 teaspoons vanilla flavor

1 cup powered sugar, sifted

Brittle

1. Preheat oven to 350.

2. Line a baking sheet with a non-stick pad.

3. In a large mixing bowl, combine quinoa, walnuts oats, chia seeds and coconut sugar.

4. Warm walnut oil and maple syrup in a small saucepan over medium heat stirring until fully incorporated.

5. Pour oil and syrup mixture over the dry ingredients, and stir to combine.

6. Pour out on non-stick baking pad, and spread into an even layer.

7. Bake for 30 minutes, turning the pan around after the first 15 minutes. Keep an eye on the brittle during the second 15 minutes to make sure it doesn't burn.

8. Let your brittle cool completely before using.

Frosting

1. Whisk all ingredients until they thicken.

2. Adjust sweetness, if necessary.

3. Refrigerate until ready for use.

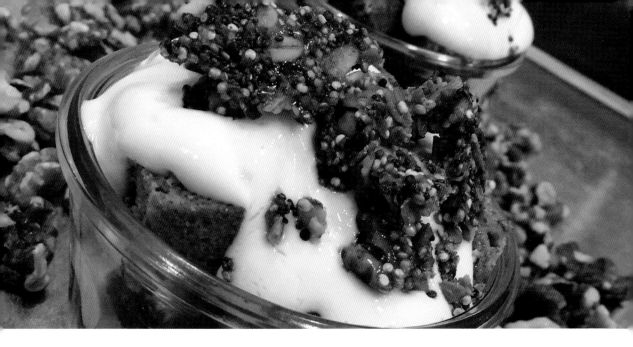

Carrot Cake

1. Preheat oven to 350.

2. Butter and flour two parchment lined nine-inch cake pans with two-inch-high sides.

3. Using electric mixer fitted with a paddle attachment, beat eggs, maple syrup and coconut oil in large bowl until smooth.

4. Add bourbon and vanilla.

5. Add in two cups of flour. Remember to scrape down the sides after each step to ensure all ingredients are well mixed in.

6. Add grated carrots, crushed pineapple and raisins.

7. In a medium bowl, combine baking soda, baking powder, salt and spices.

8. Whisk in two cups of flour to spice mixture.

9. Mix in spiced flour mixture to cake batter, and combine.

10. Pour batter into prepared pans.

11. Bake for 25 minutes, or until a toothpick inserted into center comes out clean.

12. Once the cakes are cooled, turn them out on a cutting board, and cut each cake into small squares.

13. Add some cake squares to the bottom of a Mason jar, and layer with frosting.

14. Continue this pattern. Be sure to end with a top layer of frosting.

15. Top with pieces of quinoa brittle, and finish with a drizzle of maple syrup.

Chocolate Chip Cookie and Bacon Red Velvet Waffles with Milk Chocolate Ice Cream

For Waffles

2 cups all-purpose flour

¼ cup sugar

¼ teaspoon salt

1 teaspoon baking soda

6 tablespoons unsweetened cacao powder

¼ cup butter, melted and cooled

2 cups buttermilk

3 large eggs

1 tablespoon Kahlúa

3 ounces red food coloring

6-8 slices thick apple wood smoked bacon, cooked and chopped into medium pieces (reserve some pieces for garnish)

Milk chocolate ice cream (brand of your choice)

For Cookies

2 cups all-purpose flour

½ teaspoon baking soda

1 teaspoon cinnamon

1 teaspoon salt

1 cup unsalted butter

2 cups packed brown sugar

1 ½ teaspoons vanilla extract

2 large eggs

3 cups chocolate chunks (semi-sweet, milk chocolate, or dark chocolate)

For Chocolate Sauce

8 ounces semisweet chocolate, finely chopped

1 cup heavy cream

½ cup light corn syrup

Chocolate Sauce

1. Place the chocolate in a medium bowl.

2. In a small saucepan, combine the cream and corn syrup and bring to a simmer.

3. Pour the cream mixture over the chocolate and whisk until the chocolate has melted.

4. Let your sauce cool before using.

Cookies

1. Preheat your oven to 350.

2. Combine flour, baking soda and salt in small bowl.

3. Place unsalted butter and brown sugar in the bowl of a stand mixer fitted with a paddle attachment, and beat until light and creamy.

4. Scrape the bowl to make sure all ingredients are combined.

5. Add vanilla extract and eggs, one at a time, beating well after each addition.

6. Gradually beat in flour mixture.

7. Stir in chocolate chunks.

8. Using a medium cookie scoop, place cookie dough onto silk, pad-lined baking sheets.

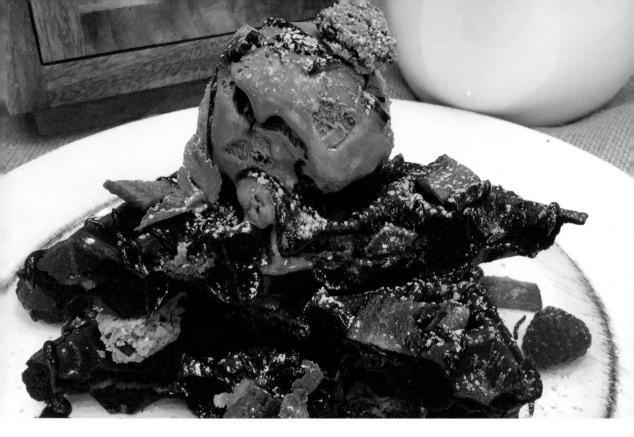

9. Bake for 12-13 minutes, or until golden brown.

10. Place cookies on wire racks to cool completely.

Red Velvet Waffles

1. Preheat your waffle iron, and spray with non-stick cooking spray.

2. Add the flour, sugar, salt, baking soda and cacao to a large mixing bowl.

3. Combine the butter, buttermilk, eggs, Kahlúa and red food coloring in a medium-mixing bowl.

4. Add the buttermilk mixture to the dry ingredients, and stir to incorporate thoroughly.

5. Spoon ¼ cup of the batter evenly onto the waffle iron and top with cookie and bacon pieces then cook until desired doneness.

6. Remove waffles as they cook, and keep warm.

7. Cut waffles in half diagonally and stack three pieces high.

8. Top with a large scoop of ice cream, and garnish with more cookie pieces, bacon, chocolate sauce, mint and fresh raspberries (optional).

Chef Richard Ingraham

Chef Richard Ingraham was born and raised in Miami, Florida and became a culinary enthusiast at an early age. His culinary training took place at the Art Institute of Atlanta.

A few years later, he was offered what is now his current position as private chef for the NBA's Dwyane Wade. He has been responsible for the diet that keeps the star fit, toned and healthy on and off the court for the past thirteen years.

In 2010, he leveraged his world-class training and passion for fine cuisine into a culinary-business partnership with Soley Gonzalez and created a network of private chefs called ChefRLI. The company has served dozens of NBA, NFL, MLB and entertainment clients across the country. Some notable current and past clients include: BET, Sean Combs, Manny Machado, John Wall, Chris Bosh, Novack Djokovic, Kelly Rowland, GOYA Foods, POMI Italia, and Blake Griffin.

In 2014, the company worked with celebrity-loved clothing line Peace Love World to create a line dedicated to foodies called Peace Love Cook.

Ingraham also joined Michelle Bernstein and Michael Schwartz in First Lady Michelle Obama's Chefs Move 2 Schools White House initiative to encourage healthier eating habits among our country's youth.

As GOYA Foods' My Plate ambassador and partner, Ingraham is also tasked with promoting alternative cooking methods to parents of school-aged children.

Chef RLI also combined its charitable efforts with Beyond the Boroughs Scholarship Fund founder and NFL vet Tutan Reyes to provide healthier eating options to kids in New York City. The Ben and Sarah Gibson Culinary Scholarship was created as a result of the partnership to help high school graduates attend culinary school.

Ingraham is also an advisory board member of the Miami Culinary Institute and Chef Start. And, he was selected for South Beach Food and Wine Festival's "The Best Thing I Ever Ate at the Beach."